THE PARENT'S GUIDE TO
COACHING PHYSICALLY CHALLENGED CHILDREN

COACHING PHYSICALLY CHALLENGED CHILDREN

BETTER
WAY
BOOKS

Richard Zulewski

CINCINNATI, OHIO

98   97   96   95   94   5   4   3   2   1

Library of Congress Cataloging-in-Publication Data

Zulewski, Richard
    The parent's guide to coaching physically challenged children / by Richard Zulewski. — 1st ed.
      p.   cm.
    Includes bibliographical references and index.
    ISBN 1-55870-347-0
    1. Sports for the handicapped—Coaching. 2. Parents of handicapped children. 3. Special Olympics. I. Title.
GV709.4.Z85 1994
790'.1'96—dc20   94-13406
                                                      CIP

Edited by Donna Collingwood
Designed by Sandy Conopeotis

This book is dedicated to my loving mother
who recently passed on to a better world.
As a nurse, fortunately for her patients,
she was years ahead of her time.
As a mother, fortunately for me,
she was years behind.

Thank you, I will always love you.

ABOUT THE AUTHOR

Richard Zulewski has been a Speech and Language Pathologist for over ten years. He has worked extensively with a variety of children who have a wide range of disabilities, speech and language problems. He also works extensively in sports training with children with physical and mental retardation. Currently he is employed by Woods Services, a year-round residential facility serving children and adults with mental and physical retardation, challenging behaviors and mental health problems, located in Langhorne, Pennsylvania.

Mr. Zulewski has previously written *The Parent's Guide to Coaching Hockey* (Betterway Books). In addition, he has written and published various newsletters on a wide range of topics for specific communities. He has also written a currently unpublished work on ice hockey simulation. Mr. Zulewski has also started his own ice hockey newspaper.

Mr. Zulewski holds a B.A. from Duquesne University in Pittsburgh, and an M.A. from Temple University in Philadelphia. He resides in Philadelphia with his wife of eight years, Kathleen, and his children, Thomas and Stephanie.

ACKNOWLEDGMENTS

Special thanks to:
The Christmann family, especially Daniel and Kevin;
The Hickey family, especially Bobby, Matthew, Kimberly and Mom, Maureen;
The Marriott family, especially Stephen, Timmy and Mom, Eileen;
The Zulewski family, especially Tommy, Stephanie and Mom, Kate, and also to:
The Speech Department: Terri Milligan, Michele Aungst, Suzanne Meier and Barbara Patton;
The Aquatics Department, especially Esther Fagan;
The Recreational Department, especially Eric Dressler, and the Staff of 356 Roebling Dr.
Thank You All

INTRODUCTION:
ALL CHILDREN ARE SPECIAL (or: FINGERS AND TOES)

The most precious gift is the gift of life. Ask any crowd of people what "the gift of life" means to them, and the images the respondents immediately concoct will be as varied as the individuals.

To many people, the idea of giving (or saving) life creates visions of that most courageous and valiant act of performing CPR on a fallen individual. To others, it may be visions of a grizzly, exhausted fire fighter, with little consideration for his own life, doing what he knows to be right and running into a burning inferno that used to be a building to rescue a helpless, fire-trapped victim.

To me the ultimate gift of life was realized when I saw my son and my daughter being born. But unlike others who perhaps take reproduction for granted, my wife and I struggled just to conceive. Each birth was a shining moment, an apex of celebration that put life and its beauty and complexity, and its simplicity and innocence, into perspective.

But, there is a significant difference in saving a life in emergency and urgent situations and in giving life to an infant. Once a fire fighter saves a life, the individuals go their own ways, with no further responsibility to each other. I've come to the realization, understanding and acceptance that the gift of life in the form of a son or daughter, however, represents a life-long commitment to quality, love and sacrifice.

This baby, this creation of life, this little bundle of joy is now, both in spirituality and responsibility, yours forever. This little package—like a good marriage: in good times and in bad, for better or for worse, in sickness and in health, until death do you part—is now your total responsibility.

But while reflecting on the events of birth, one thing struck me as very unusual. In the first few seconds after my children's births, the first thing I did—the very first thing—was count their fingers and toes. I didn't thank God for the miracle, I didn't turn to my wife to tell her I loved her, I didn't even cry with delight. "Five-five-five-five. Yup, they're all there. He's (she's) perfect!"

Later, I realized how crass I was to do such a thing. I should have been ecstatic just to have a baby, and worried about fingers and toes later. I was very disappointed in myself. After all, I'm a professional. I knew I should to be able to divorce myself from such a trivial concern, that such a small thing as a missing digit shouldn't really matter, but I did it anyway.

What was even more amazing to me, however, was what I learned in the weeks that followed. As I began to sheepishly discuss my feelings and observations with my family and peers, I realized that I wasn't alone in my actions. Just about everyone I talked to did the same thing! We all placed an artificial happiness and perfection rating on the number of toes and fingers our child had. For that moment, nothing else mattered.

In the months that followed, as my children grew, and most specifically as I began to write this book, I realized just how insensitive and downright stupid I was to do such a thing. Fingers and toes should have been the least of my worries. There are so many diseases, infirmities and afflictions that could befall my children in the years to come, that something like a missing toe seems downright ridiculous. A child could become handicapped (special, challenged, "retarded") through an accident, a fever, a fall, or a seemingly minor incident. Things we consider incidental could become devastating. But all I could do was count fingers and toes. How stupid!

One thing, however, remains constant. Regardless of what happens to my children, regardless of what they are or what they become, they will always be my children and I will always love them, come hell or high water.

If I were the parent of a special child, I would pray for strength, for devotion, and for courage to face my challenges head on. Most of all, I would pray for intelligence to be able to better understand what my wife and I could do for our child. I know we would come to the realization that we couldn't address all the needs of a special-needs child alone. We would need help—a lot of it. Help to survive, help to cope, help to educate, help to understand.

The help would likely come through mental and physical health professionals and volunteers. I would pray to find caring, loving, helpful and trustworthy individuals who know more about special needs than I do.

This book is for those volunteers, professionals, uncertain parents, coaches and others who wish to organize or participate in sports with individuals who are disabled. The book is an overview of some of the needs of special, or disabled, children. It is not comprehensive. In writing it, I hope to foster a better understanding in the uninitiated, provide a solid knowledge base and give a better insight into these wonderful individuals we call special children.

Regardless of why you are reading this book, please keep this in mind: Don't just read the words printed on the page. Take the information and live it! Apply it! Embrace it! Become a helper, a striper, a volunteer, a professional, a resource person, a teacher, a giver, a donator, a benefactor. Become a special person yourself.

Chapter One

WHAT MAKES SOME CHILDREN SPECIAL?

What makes some children special? Perhaps they have a physically or mentally handicapping condition, or they have physical or mental retardation. But what, other than a physical or mental handicap, warrants that these children be treated differently than other children?

The answer is really quite simple. There should be no difference in the way we treat or acknowledge them. We already accept as fact that there should be no difference in treatment of children of different races or religions. In fact, we know that it is illegal to treat people differently because of their religion or race. Because of the Americans With Disabilities Act, which became effective in early 1993, it is now illegal to discriminate against an individual because of physical differences also.

Special children laugh and cry and savor and hurt just like other children. They have feelings, emotions, joys and pains like everyone else. They get hungry, tired, jealous and sad. They fall in love, fall out of love, and hurt from a broken heart because of love. They get mad at people who hurt them, they like people who take care of them, they shy away from people they are unfamiliar with.

So, if all of the above is in fact true, why do we call them "special children"? Not because they are different emotionally from other children. It is not that they are visually different, although sometimes they are. Most times, you cannot tell by sight that an individual has mental retardation. The difference lies in physical and/or mental limitations. Often, exceptional children are identified only by the way they respond to the world around them or in the way they learn or fail to learn. They are individuals with special needs or who require special considerations.

Mental and/or physical limitations can include any of a wide range of characteristics. Following is a brief outline of some of the categories of mental and physical impairment and how they affect an individual. In general, special children are identified as having one or more of the following:

- sensory impairments, such as hearing or vision loss
- mental retardation
- communication disorders, such as speech and/or language disorders
- learning disabilities
- behavior disorders
- health impairments such as neurological deficiencies, orthopedic conditions, degenerative diseases, birth defects and developmental disabilities

This book will not address children with learning disabilities or behavior disorders because those two situations do not necessarily require adaptations for sports and are covered extensively in other books. We will deal with children who have mental retardation or are physically disabled. The following are some of the more common physical disabilities.

SENSORY IMPAIRMENT
Sensory impairment can mean either a hearing or a vision loss. Hearing loss in children can be caused by a number of different conditions. The condition may have originated within the developing fetus, such as genetic anomalies (called endogenous causes), or it may have been caused outside of the womb by disease or trauma (called exogenous causes).

Hearing Loss
An endogenous cause may be an inherited trait such as Treacher Collins syndrome which manifests itself in, among other things, missing or malformed external ears, auditory canals, and middle ear bones. Treacher Collins syndrome causes a conductive hearing loss. Another cause of hearing loss is Waardenburg syndrome which in-

cludes a sensorineural hearing loss. In fact, over fifty genetic syndromes have been identified as possible causes of hearing loss. Even without a diagnosed genetic cause, a child may have an inherited deafness caused by a dominant trait.

The two primary exogenous causes of hearing loss are injury and illness. For example, rubella or German measles, when contracted by the mother during the first three months of pregnancy, is a leading cause of hearing loss. Other prenatal causes of hearing loss include the mother's contraction of mumps, influenza and toxemias.

Other common causes of hearing loss at birth are prematurity, Rh incompatibility, and apnea or the inability to breathe readily during or immediately after birth.

Following birth, hearing loss can be caused by viral infections such as mumps, measles or meningitis. If left unattended for long periods of time, otitis media (or fluid accumulation in the middle ear behind the eardrum) is another common cause of hearing loss. Finally, trauma, accidents and high fevers can also be responsible for a hearing loss.

A child with a hearing loss may have significant deficiencies in speech, language and communication skills, but such a child is not significantly restricted in many activities of daily life or sports activities.

Vision Loss

On the other hand, vision loss can be devastating. Without vision, children are unable to learn in the usual way. They need to learn braille and require a reader for non-braille documents.

Sightless athletes are unable to participate in many activities. Running is difficult, and softball, volleyball, soccer and baseball are nearly impossible as it is obviously very difficult to hit or catch a moving ball that you cannot see.

There are, however, some sports that can be enjoyed by the sightless and can be adapted for better participation. A loud, constant tone echoed across the surface of the water can guide swimmers toward the pool edge. Narrow path running events can be similarly adapted. Many gymnastic activities do not require vision. Power lifting requires no sight at all. Horseback riding by vision-impaired individuals is quite common. As long as a sport can be reasonably adapted for participation without danger, it's possible for the visually impaired to enjoy it.

MENTAL RETARDATION

Mental retardation is usually classified on the following levels:

Category	Intelligence Quotient
Mild	60 − 55
Moderate	54 − 40
Severe	39 − 25
Profound	24 and below

It is difficult to adequately and accurately discuss the causes of mental retardation. More than 90 percent of mental retardation is classified as "of unknown origin." When and if the origin is determined, it is often a combination of causes.

Many instances of mental retardation are classified as mild. The causes are considered a combination of environmental conditions and inherited factors. The pathological causes include:

1. chromosomal abnormality
2. infections and intoxation
3. gross brain disease (postnatal)
4. trauma and physical agents (such as traumatic brain injury)
5. metabolism and nutrition (prenatal)
6. gestational disorders (of mother or child)
7. prenatal influence
8. psychiatric disorders

Pinpointing a specific cause of mental retardation in an individual is nearly impossible, considering the many variables that are involved. Any of the pathological factors can be present along with any of the environmental factors contributing to mental retardation.

COMMUNICATION DISORDERS

Communication disorders include a wide range of speech and language problems that affect an individual's ability to present thoughts, ideas or emotions to a listener.

Communication problems include the following:

1. Expressive or receptive vocabulary deficits
2. Expressive language deficits, including disorders of correct word usage, word structure and sentence structure
3. Receptive language problems, including deficits of understanding specific words or sentences, inability to act on or follow commands, and inability to comprehend spoken words
4. Disorders of rate or rhythm of speech, including stuttering
5. Disorders of articulation or specific production of speech sounds
6. Disorders of voice and vocal quality

The general causes for such disorders are, like causes of mental retardation, many and varied. In many cases, children have just mislearned or not learned various structures of language. Such learning might be related to poor language models in the environment, inadequate motivation, or faulty hypotheses about various language structures. These children make some mistakes in hearing, analyzing, and developing their language forms, or their environment does not provide them with appropriate examples or rewards for properly learning language. These language disorders are usually mild to moderate.

In some cases, language learning can be severely inhibited by less-than-adequate sensory perception or intellectual functioning. In these cases, the language may be severely deficient, and the child may not be able to use his language at anywhere near a satisfactory level. Children with these severe language disorders are usually classified as having mental retardation, as brain damaged, or as severely learning disabled. For whatever reasons, they have not been able to bring together the physiological and/or intellectual resources necessary to acquire language structures as complex and subtle as the ones children of similar ages have been able to acquire.

There is an important comparison between children in this category and children classified as nonspeaking. Language-disordered children, no matter how severe their problem, demonstrate an awareness that their culture has developed a formal language system which represents objects, relationships and events. Nonspeaking children do not demonstrate such an awareness. Thus, regardless of the severity of the language problem, the child who has at least some oral language and who has become a language user has demonstrated something important. He is somewhere on the normal development track. Any child who is past three or four years of age and has failed to attain this basic level is telling us that he has some severe problems in the most basic developmental areas. Chapter two more thoroughly covers communicating with special children.

LEARNING DISABILITIES

The LD label, or learning disability label, has been associated with controversy since its idealistic inception many years ago. For decades, experts could not put characteristic traits on this label to make it a complete package to sell to educators, parents or health professionals. In 1968, a breakthrough occurred when the Council for Exceptional Children (CEC) established the Division of Children with Learning Disabilities. This council helped pass legislation to institute special programs and legislative money for research, training and development. Five theoretical movements of learning disability treatments have significantly influenced the field of LD perceptual, neurological, multisensory, psycholinguistics and precision teaching.

Perceptual disorders are disorders in which children cannot read or perform because they have deficits particularly in respect to vision and visual-motor perception. *Neurological* disorders are language disorders in which the left and right sides of the brain are confused in dominance of language, the left side usually being the language dominant side. *Multisensory* disorders are those in which the combination of the senses which normally help an individual to learn are mixing their signals to the brain and the brain is equally confused as to learning.

Psycholinguistics is an admittedly vague and elusive area that communication specialists believe can affect the special child. Psycholinguistics involves the belief that learning to receive and express information is necessary before actually learning to read, write and spell. This theory, however, fails to address the child with the supposed inability to begin the process of learning, but who, nevertheless, acquires early learning skills before he or she has had an opportunity to be taught to learn. Many of the basic skills of life that relate to sports (such as walking, running, or the ability to follow simple spoken or demonstrated directions) have been acquired by children who have trouble receiving information. It remains to be determined how these skills were originally acquired and if further training in psycholinguistics is warranted, necessary or helpful.

Precision teaching follows the theory that because little can be done to aid a damaged brain, it is more important to direct attention to behaviors such as speaking, writing and walking. Furthermore, precision teachers attach little importance to underlying causes of behaviors. They tend to deal directly with the behaviors concerned.

The relationship of this subject and associated areas of learning disabilities to sports and acquiring sports skills is an elusive domain. There are many works devoted exclusively to learning disabilities available at the local library.

BEHAVIOR DISORDERS

There is no generally accepted definition of behavior disorders or of the emotionally disturbed child. A child is emotionally disturbed when someone with authority labels him or her this way. The labels are arbitrary because the definitions are not precise. People who have worked with disturbed children typically have made their own working definitions. There are a number of reasons for lack of clarity and agreement in defining behavior disorders. As with learning disabilities, the subject of behavior disorders is so vague and yet so expansive that a significant discussion of the topic is a book in itself.

Again, refer to the local library for additional information.

The problems with behavior disturbances first lie in measurement. While we can objectively measure IQ, visual acuity or auditory deficits, there are no objective tests to measure anxiety, personality or adjustment. Available tests are all subjective scales of projection that others place around the child. The child does not provide the information directly. Additionally, the child is "measured" in a sterile environment such as a psychologist's office. It is not the "real world" to the child. In the real world, the child spends time in many situations and environments and reacts according to each stimulus. In the office, spontaneity is removed.

In addition, problems lie in the lack of a clear definition of mental health. Many assume that being emotionally disturbed is the opposite of being mentally healthy. This does not add much clarity to an already muddled definition. There are some characteristics that professionals use as categorization helpers, but these are so widely varied that they create more confusion than clarification.

Differing social and cultural expectations are also contributing factors. What is an accepted standard in one household is considered abnormal or maladaptive in another. For example, children raised on the streets in a lower-class urban neighborhood may consider drug use and fighting as acceptable and possibly even normal, whereas the same situations in another neighborhood, for example a religious community, could be considered maladaptive. Conversely, the actions of individuals in the religious community may, too, be considered maladaptive by many others.

The frequency of inappropriate behaviors is the most important distinguishing feature of disturbed children. The behaviors of the disturbed child tend to be of greater or lesser intensity than those of the normal child. Finally, disturbed children usually exhibit numerous problem behaviors in more than one area of functioning.

HEALTH IMPAIRMENTS

This section covers some of the major disorders that "qualify" a child or adult as physically disabled or physically challenged. Remember, in many cases, an individual may have multiple handicaps.

While some of these physically limiting conditions are not debilitating on their own, when combined with other physical or mental challenges, these can cause significant problems.

Some of these disabilities are referred to as *acquired*; that is, they are acquired after birth rather than being present at birth, or *congenital*. This difference in onset can lead to contributing emotional and psychological factors. People with congenital disabilities sometimes have a sense of difference while those with acquired disabilities may suffer a sense of loss.

Cerebral Palsy. The largest group of physically impaired individuals have cerebral palsy. Cerebral palsy is a general category of motor handicaps that affect muscle action, coordination, strength, movement, posture, balance and skills. There are four types of cerebral palsy: spastic, athetoid, ataxic and mixed. Spastic refers to increased muscle tone; athetoid is characterized by uncontrolled, jerky and irregular movements; ataxic is a lack of coordination and balance; and mixed is a combination of the first three conditions.

Other problems associated with cerebral palsy are sensory deficits, convulsive disorders, intellectual functioning, behavior disturbances, learning and emotional coping.

Muscular Dystrophy. Muscular Dystrophy is another physical impairment. This disability causes progressive weakening of the muscular system. It is a rapidly progressive disease usually ending in death. This hereditary disorder rarely affects females.

Spina Bifida. Spina bifida occurs when a portion of the spinal cord is not enclosed by the vertebrae, causing distortion of the nerve roots and spinal cord. It eventually causes neurological disorders and related deformities. Many children with spina bifida develop an abnormal blockage or collection of cerebrospinal fluid in the cranial cavity which, if not corrected by a surgical shunt, can cause mental retardation.

Spinal Cord Injuries. Spinal cord injuries are usually a result of trauma such as an automobile, swimming or bicycle accident. They result in paraplegia or quadriplegia. Potential problem areas include urinary tract infections, respiratory infections, pressure sores from lack of movement and mobility problems.

Limb Deficiencies. Limb deficiencies can be acquired or congenital and present a major obstacle to function and physical activity. Early intervention is crucial to get maximum benefit from rehabilitative therapy. An individual may or may not choose to use an artificial limb. Psychological problems related to the disability are quite common.

Juvenile Rheumatoid Arthritis. JRA is a chronic inflammatory disease of the joints and the tissues around them. Fever spikes, rash and morning stiffness are characteristic symptoms that often result in absences from school and other activities. Children with JRA need freedom of movement and may require adaptive equipment to complete daily activities.

Epilepsy. Epilepsy, or seizure disorder, can be a problem entirely to itself or may be associated with many other disorders. Seizures are caused by abnormal or excessive electrical brain discharges. Not all seizures are readily visible. Seizure intensity may be either grand mal or petit mal. Grand mal seizures are easily recognized by falling to the ground and/or violent shaking of the body, while many petit mal seizures go unnoticed by even the most discriminating observer. Seizures can be controlled and managed by medication; however, heavy medication may seriously affect learning, performance and personality. It should be noted that alteration of the brain function associated with seizure disorder does not imply associated learning disorders. Many individuals with seizure disorder live normal and completely unaffected lives.

Juvenile Diabetes Mellitus. Juvenile diabetes mellitus is an often hereditary metabolic disorder characterized by the body's inability to convert sugars and starches to energy. The pancreas does not produce enough insulin, and sometimes injections are necessary. A child may react to either too much or not enough insulin. The symptoms of insulin deficiency, or ketoacidosis, include onset of fatigue, drinking large amounts of water, producing large amounts of urine, excessive hunger, deep breathing and/or warm, dry skin. The symptoms of insulin excess, or insulin reaction, include rapid onset of headache, nausea, vomiting, palpitations, irritability, shallow breathing, and/or cold, moist skin.

Hemophilia. Hemophilia, or "bleeder's disease," is rarely found in females. It is characterized by poor blood clotting ability. What may cause only a bump or bruise normally can cause severe internal bleeding in the hemophiliac. This bleeding can cause accumulation of blood in the joints causing temporary immobility and pain.

Cystic Fibrosis. Cystic fibrosis is a hereditary disorder characterized by chronic lung (pulmonary) disease, pancreatic deficiency, and high levels of sweet electrolytes, which causes a serum-like sweat. Respiratory symptoms, including a dry, nonproductive cough, susceptibility to acute infection, and bronchial obstruction by abnormal secretions, are major problems.

Sickle Cell Anemia. Sickle cell anemia is a hereditary disorder prevalent in, but not limited to, African-Americans. The sickle-shaped cells do not pass easily through the blood vessels and may suddenly cut off blood supply to some tissues, causing severe pain in the abdomen, legs and arms; swelling of the joints; fatigue and high fever.

Heart Conditions. Heart (cardiac) conditions may be congenital or acquired. If acquired, they usually are the result of an infectious disease such as rheumatic fever. Congenital defects may not appear or be detected until later in life and may be assumed to be acquired.

Cancer. Cancer is an uncontrolled irregular cell growth of unknown origin. In children, leukemia and tumors of the eyes, brain, bone and kidney are most common. Side effects of the disease and treatment include emotional problems, fatigue, extreme weight loss or gain, nausea, susceptibility to upper respiratory infections, headaches and baldness.

This assortment of childhood health impairments or causes of mental or physical retardation is not all-inclusive. They are merely the most common and recognizable of the multitude of mental or physical health problems that can afflict children and directly affect their quality of life.

Regardless of the physical or mental problems a child may have, it is extremely important to get reliable medical approval before his or her participation in any exercise, exercise-related or physical activity program. For coaches, it is helpful, if possible, to ask a child's physician for limits, exclusions and/or recommendations concerning that child. No one, however, other than a child's parents or legal guardians (preferably after consultation with the child's personal physician), should approve that child's participation in any physical activity.

Despite the physical and mental differences discussed in this chapter, most of these children are like any others. Regardless of what you want to call them—special, disabled, retarded, physically challenged—you still call them children. They possess the full range of emotions, feelings, passions and sensations. Keep this foremost in your mind as you work with special children, whether as a coach, therapist, volunteer or concerned parent: If you treat each child as you would expect to be treated—with respect, consideration and love—you can expect the same in return.

Chapter Two

COMMUNICATING WITH SPECIAL CHILDREN

Think back to the time you last went to a foreign country (Canada doesn't count unless it was the province of Quebec). You probably didn't speak the language. Getting around was difficult, but certainly not impossible. Using all your street smarts and savvy, you employed a conglomeration of broken foreign phrases, body language, gestures, pointing, and maybe even some kind of communication help book to get you through the rough times.

To get your hands on a big Mc-something-or-other for lunch, one thing you might have done was to show pictures of the big *M*. Perhaps, you made eating motions with your hands and made yourself look hungry or quizzical when you asked for directions. In return, the not-so-lucky passerby whom you stopped for directions was at an equal disadvantage with your language. Realizing you were a foreigner and hopefully following your lead, your helper began by using short phrases containing simple words in the native tongue. If that didn't work, gestures, pointing, and extended fingers served to show how many blocks you had to travel.

The most important thing to you, however, was that your method — regardless of how crude and simplistic — worked and you got to fill your stomach! It may have been a difficult and somewhat laborious process, but it worked!

As your time in the country lengthened, you gained proficiency in the language simply out of necessity. You began to better find your way around the city as you could read and understand street signs and directions. If you stayed long enough, you eventually were able to get along on your own with little help. It was nothing to stop and ask strangers any type of question, because you felt more comfortable and adept in dealing with the language. In a very short time, as a matter of survival, you became masterful and skillful with the language.

Practically speaking, there is no real difference between learning a foreign language and learning the language of our parents. To take it one step further, the process is similar for special children trying to learn our language. But special children usually take longer to learn the language, or they must be instructed in a different manner than is customary.

RECEPTIVE AND EXPRESSIVE LANGUAGE

Communicatively, two types of language are employed in everyday conversation. When special educators and communication specialists speak of language, they don't speak of English, Spanish or French. They speak of *expressive* and *receptive* language. Expressive language is used by a speaker taking thoughts, ideas and emotions in the brain and expressing these thoughts by transforming them into recognizable sounds known as a voice.

Expressive language is also accompanied by the visual output that speakers use to emphasize their message. Speakers' hand gestures, facial expressions, grimaces and body language accompany their speech and embellish their message. Very few people have a flat effect in communicating, that is, no expression, no vocal inflection, no gestures.

Receptive language is used by a listener taking in the sounds of the spoken voice, transforming the sounds into mechanical energy in the middle ear, then sending electrical impulses from the inner ear to finally create brain waves that the brain perceives as sound. (Of course, the process is significantly more complicated than this, but this is just to serve an illustrative purpose.) Receptive language is also accompanied and embellished by the speaker's visual presentation that the listener takes into consideration when determining the message.

For example, when discovering that your three-year-old son has just colored a big purple dinosaur on the dining room wall, you most certainly will call out his name in frustration to summon him.

"Tommy!" But just calling his name is not enough. To express the urgency and frustration of the situation, you might say it with elevated volume, with emphasis, with frustration, and with your hands on your hips. "T-O-M-M-Y!" When your son finally shows up at the scene of the crime, he knows he's in deep trouble without any more being said. The toddler, looking at Mom's or Dad's glaring face, receives a very distinct message. The child, eyes filling with tears, draws back from the scene, which also says a lot. A significant communication exchange is going on without a lot of speech.

Transmitting expressive and receptive language is what constitutes communication. Communication expresses feelings, ideas and information, and, as we have seen, it does not necessarily mean all spoken or verbal output. As long as a message is transmitted between two persons, communication is taking place. Communication exists in many forms: facial expressions, body language, gestures, speech, sign language, written language and pictures.

COMMUNICATION DEVELOPMENT IN THE SPECIAL CHILD

In our everyday world, communication takes place constantly. The general population uses spoken language, the deaf population uses sign language, and the severe to profound population uses a series of grunts, sounds, meaningful and meaningless noises, cries, facial expressions or combinations of these to communicate.

We as parents, coaches and volunteers need to know and understand some of the simple milestones of normal communication and how they relate to special children. At six months, babies begin to coo, gurgle, and inflect tones in their voices. At one year, an infant may begin to use familiar simple words, such as *mama* for mommy, *wawa* for water, or any of the other simplistic or repetitive words we know as baby talk. At two years, toddlers begin to put together meaningful phrases of two to three words, and by three years, they are using simple but complete sentences.

With the special child population, we need to be aware of two specific numbers that are often associated with cognitive levels of functioning. You will hear age referred to as chronological age (known as the CA), designated in years and months if the child is older (expressed as for example 5 years, 2 months; 5y,2m; 5-2 or 5.2) or designated in total months if the child is younger (such as 15 months or 15m). You will then hear about perceived or tested mental age (known as the MA) indicated the same way as chronological age.

A child with a chronological age of fifteen years does not necessarily have a mental age of fifteen years. Mentally, the child may be functioning at the two- or three-year-old level. Parents, coaches and volunteers need to speak to such a child as they would speak to a two- or three-year-old child and not as they would to a fifteen-year-old child. That does *not* mean to talk down to the child and use baby talk. It means to use simple, basic vocabulary; simple sentence structure and simple commands; and not complex, sophisticated words. Keep in mind that the child needs to have receptive language skills to process the information.

Simplify Whenever Possible

Use simple language structure in any situation even if a child just has mental retardation. In many situations, a child may have additional problems that compound expressive or receptive language difficulties. Along with retardation, a child may also have a learning disability, be brain injured, have a hearing loss, have cerebral palsy, or have any combination of these problems. The communication problems with the special child are then magnified one, two or three times.

An example of simple language is saying "My car's broken and needs fixing" rather than "My car is in disrepair and needs attending to." A coach may be apt to say something like "Strike the ball sharply and toward the gap in left-center." Replace that with "Hit it hard that way." The messages in both cases are identical. However, one message was complicated with extraneous words while the other was short, simple and to the point.

The goal for any child with a communication difficulty, and not necessarily just those children with special difficulties, is to develop the most functional and appropriate communication possible. What this means is that two children with similar diagnoses, ages and physical appearances may not have similar communication techniques, strategies or abilities. What works for one child may not work for another child because they may not have similar communication deficits.

The parent or coach of a special child needs to be adaptable to the wide range of communication abilities of the child. When giving instructions to a child, the teacher, parent, instructor or coach needs to be aware of the problems that a child faces, and should try to understand the needs of the children under his or her tutelage and adapt as necessary to fill those needs. Remember: Simplify your language but don't use baby talk; simplify your words but don't use baby words.

Caregivers may also be called on to care for or instruct children who have severe or profound mental retardation and should be aware of some of the skills a child needs to fully benefit from interactive communication. A child must have certain prelinguistic skills to fully benefit from instruction. These prelinguistic skills include:

- attending to a situation or speaker (looking at the speaker) with more than fleeting eye contact
- awareness of the environment (looking around the room or location)
- visual tracking skills (following a moving object across the field of vision)
- auditory awareness of a speaker or noise (reacting to or startling at loud noises and voices)
- auditory localization (turning head or shifting eyes toward a sound)
- motor or verbal imitation (following simple gestures and hand movements, imitating simple facial expressions like sticking out the tongue, or attempting to imitate sounds)
- vocalization (cooing, gurgling, babbling)

Most, but certainly not all, of these skills are or should be present as a child reaches the six-month mental age level. Some skills will begin to emerge earlier, while others will emerge much later and possibly not at all. When most of these prelinguistic skills are present in a special child, we know that that child is ready to be instructed in any of the habilitative disciplines.

Following is a compiled guide to language learning that parents should know and understand. Although it is comprehensive, it is by no means complete. It is meant simply as a primer in learning to communicate with special children.

GUIDELINES FOR COMMUNICATING WITH THE SPECIAL CHILD

Remember: You are a teacher at all times. Speech and language are functions that we never stop learning. Teach not only words, skills and sports, but also essential developmental skills that will benefit a child.

Talk to the child. Infants may not seem to understand, but remember, they first learn to understand before they learn to speak. Also, remember the learning differences between expressive and receptive language skills.

Encourage any attempts to communicate. When a child seems to have no language, encourage babbling, gesturing or using a combination of sign language and gestures. Whatever speech or communication sparks an interest should be encouraged through repetition so that an awareness of and interest in communication can develop. Praise all attempts the child makes.

Reinforce spoken language. If gesture or sign language is the child's only form of communication, accept this but reinforce spoken language by verbalizing the child's needs or thoughts; however, do not accept gestures if you are sure the child knows how to speak. If a child has trouble expressing himself or herself, say it yourself and have the child repeat it. Accept both speech and gesture.

Make speaking a positive experience. The speech or communication situation should be a pleasant experience for the child. Show pleasure in conversation and let children know that you are pleased at their communication attempts by smiling at them or verbally praising them for any communication effort. If they ask for something, try to get it for them as soon as possible to demonstrate to them that communication and language have meaning.

Talk, talk, talk! Talk as much as possible about anything and everything. Talk to the child while you are preparing to participate in an activity, idly standing there waiting for an event to begin, or just watching. Talk while you are eating, walking, or even just observing the child. Explain what you are doing, what the child is doing, where you are and where you are going, and talk specifically about the activity you are involved in.

Encourage awareness of suroundings. For children who can talk, ask them to describe things they see or hear, to talk about what they're doing, or to explain the activity or sport so you are confident they know what is expected of them.

Be a good listener. If the child doesn't talk well, be patient and listen to what he or she is asking or saying. Be straightforward and tell the child that you do not understand him or her, but you'll keep trying. Do not forget that a discouraging look on your face can be as damaging as an impatient or unkind word.

Keep your language short and simple. Pronounce your words clearly when the child is facing you. Provide a good, clear speech model.

Give one direction at a time. Do not confuse the child. One direction may simply be addressing a child and asking him to go somewhere. An apparently simple direction such as: "John, go over to the new coach and ask him when the event starts, then come back here" is actually a complex of four directions. Choose your words carefully. You may need to break down extensive communication into smaller parts so the child can understand it fully.

Be patient. If you ask a question, allow sufficient time for the child to respond. The length of response will vary from individual to individual. Do not anticipate needs so that the child feels no need to communicate.

Use repetition. Repetition is necessary for language learning and understanding, so do not hesitate to reread or retell stories, directions, instructions or encouragement. You might need to repeat directions or statements three, four or five times before an individual understands the communication. Do not repeat the same statement the same way each time. Restate the directions slightly differently each time. You may use "John, it's time to go" or "Let's go, John" or "Come on, John, it's time to go" or just "Let's go." The message content remains the same while the message delivery is changed.

Encourage different responses. When communicating with a nonverbal child who has a physical disability, it is important to encourage and reinforce all types of responsive behaviors, such as a smile, a frown, a head nod, a hand raise or even a seemingly aggressive response such as grabbing or yelling. It may be that child's only way of responding and reacting to your statement.

Assume that children understand. Don't say anything in their presence that you wouldn't want them to hear. A child may have a more intact receptive language ability along with a more impaired expressive language ability. Some children appear lower functioning than they really are.

Make sure you are consistent. Your speech and body language, facial expressions and gestures should work together. Do not give mixed signals.

AUGMENTATIVE COMMUNICATION DEVICES

Guidelines for communicating with nonverbal children using augmentative communication devices are slightly different from those just described. An augmentative communication device is a manufactured system of communication that is a substitute for or a supplement to a person's natural communication ability or skill. An augmentative communication device can be something as simple as a three-picture direct select language communication board or as complicated as an advanced multilevel electronic talking device.

Language boards or devices are used in a variety of settings for a variety of reasons. A language board is usually a laminated poster board sheet of varying size with a set style of pictures arranged purposefully on it. A person uses the board to construct a message to a listener by pointing to selected pictures, in a specific and comprehensive order, to create a sentence. It is another form of expressive language.

With an electronic language board or device the individual uses the same basic selecting procedures, but the device electronically "says" the message or selected words instead of having the listener read the pictures. An electronic device user may use a switch to activate a scan of the pictures if he is unable to use his fingers or hands.

The primary reason for using an augmentative device is that a child is nonverbal. Do not, however, confuse nonverbal with unintelligent or uncommunicative. A child may be nonverbal for any number of reasons, including athetoid cerebral palsy (the most common reason) and amyotrophic (diminished) vocal chords among other things. A child who cannot speak still has something to say. Most children who are nonverbal have just as much to convey as speaking individuals; they just do not have as much opportunity to express themselves as verbal individuals do.

When using an augmentative device with a nonverbal individual, some guidelines should be followed to make using the device more pleasurable and complete for the speaker and the listener.

Guidelines for Using Augmentative Communication Devices

Access is important. The communication device should be accessible to the individual at all times and in good condition or working order so that he or she can initiate communication throughout the day. Make sure it is turned on if it is electronic. If you do not know how to turn it on or maintain it, ask someone who does know to at least show you the basics.

Encourage use. When communicating, encourage the child to use the board or device at all times. Do not rely only on yes/no responses and don't use the "twenty questions" approach to communication. Rely on yes/no only if that is the sole means of communication for the individual. Be patient!

Don't anticipate needs. Encourage the child to communicate basic wants and needs using the communication device or board. Do not anticipate children's needs before they have had the opportunity to express themselves unless it is in the normal realm of your duties.

Make your communications and interactions as meaningful as possible. If a child asks for a drink, try to get the drink as soon as possible. Show the child that communication can cause actions and effects.

Provide opportunities for the individual to communicate casually. For example, you could say something like "Wow, did you see that? What do you think about that? What do you think he'll do next? What would you do next?"

Ask appropriate questions to aid in communication. You can ask "Is it on your board?" or "Is it about _____?" to gain a better focus on communication.

Be observant. Learn how each individual indicates that he or she has something to say. Different children with similar problems may communicate in different manners. Each child may use certain movements, vocalizations, pointing, eyeing numbers for a number encoding board, or any innovative method that works.

Ask questions that require using the board. Try "When do you go home next?" as opposed to "Are you going home this weekend?" The first requires an interactive response while the second requires only one word.

Encourage verbalization. If the individual has some speech skills, encourage verbalizing in addition to using the board. If the child has significant speech skills, use the board only as a supplemental device to augment unintelligible or unrecognizable speech.

Provide choices. Give the individual two or three choices so that decisions only require processing short bits of information. Don't ask for a long explanation about something when a short, simple response will suffice. For example, the question "Do you want water, milk or juice?" is sufficient and provides the appropriate choices.

Set aside a period of time whenever you have contact with the child to work on specific communication skills related to the events of the day. Coordinate this work with any speech therapy the individual may be receiving. Don't be afraid to ask professionals for additional hints or suggestions to communicate better with the child.

Be patient! Wait for the child to process and respond. Communication using a language board takes longer than verbal communication. Don't try to guess a person's message. Repeat the individual's message aloud to ensure that you have understood what he or she is trying to communicate and to provide verbal feedback to the child to check against for accuracy.

Let the speech therapist know if the existing vocabulary is appropriate or if the child needs new pictures or words. What is adequate at one point in time or place is not necessarily acceptable in all situations.

Inform others in the child's environment (such as volunteers and other children) that the child has a language board, and show how it is used. Keep the language board free from other materials and obstructions. Make sure the entire board is visible to the individual at all times. Make sure the boards are transported back and forth with the child at all times. When we speak, we don't leave our voice at one spot. A language board is a "voice" for the person. The child needs to have it always. Remember that the communication device is the individual's primary means of communication and may be the only means. When people only have a yes/no response, they have no means of initiating communication without the board or device.

Suggested Maintenance Tips for Communication Devices

• When it is not in use (at night, during swimming, etc.), keep the board or device in a safe place.

• The Plexiglas, glycine or laminate used to protect a language board should be kept clean and in good repair at all times. Wipe up spills immediately.

• When a board is being transported in the rain or snow, provide a protective covering of plastic or other waterproof fabric. Particularly, make sure that you protect an electronic device completely at all times.

• Remember that electronic boards need to be charged periodically. If you have the opportunity, charge the device while the child is not using it, such as at night or during nap time.

• Remember that electronic devices are delicate and costly. Handle them with the utmost care.

- Never open an electronic device to see how it works or attempt to repair it. Devices should be sent back to the factory for repairs.
- Contact a speech-language pathologist or other communication professional if you suspect the device is not functioning properly.

SIGN LANGUAGE

Sign language is a form of *total communication*, a philosophy that advocates using any and all means of communication to provide unlimited opportunity for language development. Included in the total communication approach are the following: speech, hearing aids, speech reading, gesturing, signs, finger spelling, reading, writing, pictures, and any other possible means of conveying ideas, language and vocabulary. Using total communication is now the standard procedure for many individuals who have mental retardation.

Sign language is a complete language in itself, not a form of augmentative communication. Sign language generally is the means of communication in individuals of average intelligence with a hearing impairment. For individuals with mental retardation, however, sign language is used as a supplement to communication. Many individuals with mental retardation have good or even excellent hearing. Sign language is used to supplement the spoken or expressive language to help establish the message. In addition, it is easier to read and understand a message when it is accompanied by sign language.

History

The language of signs and finger spelling was brought to America from France in the early nineteenth century. In 1815, a group of men from Hartford, Connecticut, became interested in establishing a school for deaf children but lacked information on the proper means of educating the deaf. One of these gentlemen, Dr. Mason Cogswell, was particularly interested because his daughter, Alice, was deaf and had been taught on an experimental basis by a young minister, Dr. Thomas Hopkins Gallaudet. Dr. Gallaudet spent several months in Europe studying educational methods in sign language as well as the signs themselves. Soon he was ready to return to America. He established the first permanent school for the deaf in Hartford, Connecticut, in 1817.

His dream of a university for deaf students was realized when his son, Edward Miner Gallaudet, established Gallaudet College, the world's first and only college for deaf students, located in Washington, D.C. The college was chartered in 1864 by president Abraham Lincoln.

Universality

It is often wondered if sign language is universal. Certainly its use extends across the boundaries of many countries, but each country has developed its own system. In recent years, an international sign language has been developed that crosses national barriers and permits communication among deaf persons of many countries. This is useful for events such as Special Olympics International. It is also known that people who understand the language of signs find they can communicate with deaf people across language barriers more easily than is possible with hearing persons using spoken languages.

In certain educational settings in the United States, proficiency in sign language is used to fulfill a language requirement at the university level. Sign language is also looked upon by many as a new art form and is used in performances by the National Theater for the Deaf, a professional drama group, as a means of presenting deaf people and their language to a hearing world.

Since the Americans With Disabilities Act (ADA) was passed by Congress in early 1992 and became effective in early 1993, many companies are required to provide sign language interpreters either for their employees or their customers. This trend is expected to continue.

Types

In the United States, there are two similar types, or schools, of sign language in use. The most common sign language system is American Sign Language (ASL). The second and less common system is Signing Exact English (SEE). The two systems share about

90 percent of their signs, but there is that 10 percent of signs that occasionally confuses people.

ASL is a gesture-based system that develops some signs in an arbitrary or random manner. SEE bases its signs on customary and commonsense gestures that developed over the years. ASL is the most commonly used and taught system in the United States. It has a very extensive vocabulary.

SEE is used more extensively in facilities with individuals with mental retardation. Because it is generally considered easier to learn and use, and is more common sense based, SEE is easier for individuals with mental retardation to learn or understand. Unfortunately, SEE does not have the extensive vocabulary that ASL has, nor is it taught in workshops, community colleges and night schools. When people think of sign language, they automatically think of ASL.

Finger spelling. Finger spelling, or using hand positions to represent letters of the alphabet, is much older than the language of signs. It is sometimes used to supplement ASL or SEE. The positions of the fingers of the hand do, to some extent, resemble the printed letters of the alphabet. Even as early as the tenth century, monks of the Middle Ages used finger spelling as a means of communication. Today, each country has a manual alphabet which uses its own versions and is therefore only understood by users of that particular system.

It is important to remember that, regardless of the method chosen to teach or follow, there are basic, fundamental guidelines that need to be followed. These guidelines are universal to all individuals in any setting. Do not be concerned about the differences of the signs between ASL and SEE. Regardless of the system of use, if you use enough correct signs of either system in the correct context, the message will be clear even with gaps in sentence structure. Remember, in dealing with individuals with multiple handicaps, sign language is used as a supplement to spoken communication and not entirely as a communication system. The spoken words and accompanying expressive language will help fill in the gaps.

Guidelines for Communicating With Sign Language

Keep signing simple. When signing to an individual, it is best to sign only the meaningful words although you speak the entire sentence. For example, you might say "Come on, it's time to eat" but sign only "time-eat"; or say "Go to the bathroom" but sign only "go-bathroom."

Provide a good model. Speak in grammatically complete sentences, not in staccato telegraphic sentences, but sign only key words. Signs should be made in front of the body and should be clearly visible. The individual will use you and your presentation as a future model.

Build the sign vocabulary. It is often appropriate to sign words that a child may not use yet. An individual needs to see signs being used so he or she understands them as a communication system or system supplement.

Be consistent in the signs you use. Signs should be made the same way by others who communicate with the individual. Also, be consistent in the methodology of signs used. Find out whether the child knows ASL or SEE signs. Although most of the signs are equivalent, there are differences that may confuse the child.

Make your signs smoothly and steadily. Speak in a normal tone of voice. Do not yell or speak too loudly; neither should you whisper or mouth the words.

Complement your signs. Use appropriate facial expressions and body language to go with what you are signing. Signs can be emphasized in the same way spoken words can.

Encourage and inform. Encourage as many people as possible to sign with the individual so he or she doesn't associate communication with just one person. Inform others (volunteers, coaches, judges) of the extent of the child's signing and what he or she can or will sign. When possible, let children who sign demonstrate the signs to others. Although you should always use accurate signs, don't expect perfectly signed responses from the individual. Gradually shape the responses.

Ways to encourage an individual to sign

- Ask an appropriate question (for example, "What do you want?").
- Provide choices as often as possible to encourage functional communication (for example, "Do you want milk or juice?" or "Do you want to watch baseball or running?").
- Remind and encourage the individual to sign.
- Provide the appropriate verbal and sign model.
- Use hand-over-hand assistance to shape the individual's sign if necessary.

As you can see, special children are often special in more than just one way. The multitude of problems and challenges that special children present requires parents and coaches to give individual instruction and coaching.

HEARING AIDS

There is one final consideration for communication with special children: a hearing loss as determined by a qualified audiologist either unaided or corrected/supplemented by a hearing aid.

Hearing Classifications

A hearing test in a sound-dampening booth by an audiologist is used to test hearing acuity. Hearing losses are classified by the number of decibels a sound must be raised in volume (loudness) to bring the hearing to "normal." It must be noted that zero decibels is not the complete absence of sound but the very least amount of sound that a person with normal hearing acuity can hear.

The classifications and loss amounts are as follows:

Classifications	Decibel Loss
Normal	0–30 decibels
Mild	31–45 decibels
Moderate	46–60 decibels
Severe	61–75 decibels
Profound	greater than 75 decibels

To correct a common misconception, a hearing aid does not improve a person's hearing. All a hearing aid really does is consume the sound presented to the built-in microphone and then amplify it directly into the affected ear through a fully inserted ear mold. When a child uses a hearing aid, there are also precautions and guidelines for its use.

Like any electronic device, a hearing aid is sensitive to moisture, water and abuse. Care for the aid as you would any other communication device. Keep it clean and protected at all times. Wipe it off with a clean cloth if water, perspiration or rain contacts it. Do not let children swim while wearing a hearing aid.

Reminders for Dealing With Hearing Aids

Make sure the battery is fresh. Check the battery at the beginning of the day by removing the aid from the ear, turning up the volume, and cupping the aid in the hands to produce squealing feedback. If you hear a loud whistling, then the battery is functioning well. If you do not hear it, replace the battery and try again. If it still does not whistle, the tubing to the ear mold or the ear mold itself may be clogged with wax. If necessary, remove the ear mold and tubing by unscrewing them from the hearing aid, and clean them with warm soapy water. If it still does not work, it is probably broken.

Keep a supply of batteries handy at all times. The most common cause of a nonfunctioning hearing aid is a dead battery. All hearing aid batteries are now zinc-air batteries. They do not die gradually like the old mercury batteries, but die suddenly and completely. It is entirely possible that a battery may be working in the morning when you first test it but not in the afternoon or evening after a long day of use.

For each child who wears a hearing aid, know the type of battery required, how to change the battery, what volume setting is appropriate, and what ear the aid is for. The hearing aid is not changeable to opposite ears or to different individuals. It was manufactured and set to a particular ear. Hearing aids are custom adjusted and the ear molds are custom designed for the individual. You cannot take a hearing aid from one individual and put it on another.

Like a communication device or your own hearing, you should not leave the hearing aid behind. The participant should be wearing it at all times unless in a program that doesn't allow it. He has a right to hear what is going on and being said to him without difficulty.

When speaking to an individual who wears a hearing aid, speak in your normal tone and volume. The aid will compensate for the loss of hearing so it isn't necessary to raise your voice. It is still preferable, however, to stand in the wearer's line of sight so he can read your body language and facial expressions; you may be supplementing the communication with sign language. If an individual has a profound hearing loss, the aid may not be powerful enough to bring the sound up to normal volume and may be used for sound awareness only.

Be aware of the three types of hearing aids: an in-the-ear (ITE) aid which fits completely inside the ear, a behind-the-ear (BTE) aid which hangs over the rear of the ear, and a body aid which resembles a small transistor radio and is usually clipped to a front shirt pocket. Become familiar with the characteristics of each aid.

Keep in mind the following precautions:

• Do not leave the aid where it can become overheated or damaged, such as in direct sunlight or on a heat source.

• Do not drop the aid. It must be handled like the sensitive electronic instrument that it is.

• Do not bend, twist or snag the cord, tubes or ear molds, battery draws or dials. These parts are easily broken when not cared for.

• Take the batteries out of the aid when it will not be used for an extended period of time, such as for a few days.

• For a body aid, keep a spare cord handy. Replace the cord when the sound cuts off and on. The cord is the most vulnerable part of a body aid and is the most likely cause of malfunction.

• Clean the earpiece with soap and warm water when it becomes dirty or wax filled. Make sure it is dry and all the soap and water are blown out of the holes before putting it back onto the aid.

• Each time the hearing aid is worn, be sure the earpiece is firmly and correctly seated in the ear and the volume of the hearing aid is not on full gain (maximum volume) in order to prevent feedback squealing and further hearing damage.

• If you detect a problem that you cannot readily fix, contact a speech therapist or hearing aid specialist. Do not open the aid and attempt to fix it yourself.

This chapter should be considered a comprehensive primer for parents and coaches and an aid in initiating beneficial and meaningful conversation. There are so many variances and peculiarities in any individual's communication abilities that one person cannot know, fully understand and follow them all. What this chapter has attempted to do is provide a wide range of most-likely scenarios that a parent or coach may encounter in everyday meetings.

The most important key to understanding communication with an individual who has impaired abilities is to not be afraid to ask. Unless you are the one individual who has worked with a child for most of his life (not likely unless you are the parent) *and* you are the person who has developed his communication system (possible, but again not likely), then you can only learn more about the child by conversing with and asking questions of those who are familiar with that child.

Whom to ask for advice may be your biggest stumbling block. The first person to ask about the child is the primary caregiver. It is that person who spends the most time with the special child, and it is that person from whom you can most benefit.

You can gain additional knowledge and skills by asking, and conversely, the special children improve their skills from your better understanding of them. You are able to better help them meet their goals and objectives as you become more proficient in communicating with them.

Chapter Three

GENERAL EXERCISES AND MOVEMENTS

Before anyone, regardless of physical development or mental ability, begins an exercise program, two important items must be covered. First, any exercises or programs must be approved by a physician. This is especially true for the special child. By no means should a parent allow a child who is limited physically and/or mentally to begin a strenuous or even a leisurely stretching or exercise program without first examining all the ramifications of the program. Let a physician help determine if the advantages outweigh the disadvantages. Something that is or should be a simple maneuver for a non-challenged child may be too complicated or too dangerous for a child with a physical retardation or limitation.

Second, it is important to exercise with a realistic goal in mind. It is not feasible to expect the child to accomplish twenty or thirty repetitions of an exercise when just initiating a workout regimen. A better goal for any individual is to achieve and maintain overall body fitness with exercises that require stretching , relaxing, flexing and moving muscles as much as possible without overdoing it and to maintain this level rather than increase it. If it's important to increase the number of repetitions, it should be done in small increments. If everyone else is doing twenty repetitions of an exercise and the child can only do seven, he should do seven repetitions that are good, complete and appropriate. It's better to do seven or even five than none at all.

It isn't necessary to stretch and exercise every single day. Research shows that exercising at least every other day will cause a major change. That's not a bad schedule to keep and one that is easy to maintain.

Most of the exercises described in this chapter can be done standing up, sitting down or even lying down so individuals in wheelchairs have equal opportunity to exercise. Other than the physical limitations placed by the physician, there is no reason not to do them. Some of the exercises are rather easy. Some are minimally difficult but doable and others may prove to be too strenuous for some individuals. The second the child starts feeling stress, cease activity immediately. I'm not talking about the stiffness or mild aching experienced when first starting an exercise program. I refer to serious discomfort and pain. This is what you need to be concerned about.

Keep accurate records or notes of the exercises. Record the type of exercise performed, the number of movements per repetition, and the number of repetitions per sitting. If the child does five of something for a week, the next week have her try six. This is not asking too much; in fact it should result in better ability to perform the exercises.

Four types of exercises are employed in this section: warm-up, isometric (pushing against a stationary object), isotonic (moving a weighted object) and cooling-down exercises. Although these terms may be new to you, the exercises will not be new. They are all variations of exercises that you have performed before. I have grouped them into categories to make them easy to remember and perform.

The exercises are grouped according to type of exercise and then are ordered from the head down to the toes. By following the exercises in the order presented, the body is systematically stretched and exercised in a logical and complete order. Also, by following this type of exercise progression, the body moves from stretching to slightly more difficult work to yet harder work and finally back to relaxation. There is a logical flow to the progression of the exercises and the body is worked out without undue stress.

It is important to begin each exercise session with deep breathing techniques. The body and the muscles need oxygen to function properly. Without oxygen, the muscles will begin to cramp.

WARM-UP EXERCISES

Breathing: Straighten back, close mouth, and breathe in through the nose. Attempt to fill the lungs as much as possible. Look down to watch the chest begin to expand. Avoid filling the stomach by pulling in and down on the diaphragm. Filling the stomach with air has no benefits. The stomach does not and cannot convey the oxygen into the blood stream and if the stomach becomes distended (filled with air) it will be very uncomfortable. The stomach *may* inflate a *little* as the diaphragm pushes it down and out of the way and the lungs fill with air, but it should never enlarge greatly. Never hold the breath for longer than one second. Finally, exhale the air slowly through the mouth and over the lips. Pull in the stomach to expel all residual air. Repeat up to five times to begin.

Head tilts: Slowly bend the head left and right to opposite shoulders and then return to starting position. Do not twist and turn the head. A continuation or variation of this move is to tilt the head forward toward the chest and then backward looking straight up, alternating movements. Repeat as able for up to five times.

Head rolls: Slowly rotate or roll the head around the shoulders to stretch the muscles. Do this for up to one-half minute.

Shoulder shrugs: To strengthen neck muscles, shrug the shoulders tightly, hold for a count of five and then drop them to normal position. Repeat up to five times.

Shoulder stretches: Interlock fingers in front of the chest, turn the palms out away from the chest and slowly straighten the elbows and lift the arms overhead. Stretch as far as possible without pain. Hold for a count of five and repeat up to five times.

Shoulder touches: Lift arms straight up overhead with palms in, then bend the elbows and touch the shoulders with the fingertips. Repeat up to five times.

Arm stretches: To strengthen shoulder muscles and increase circulation, straighten the arms down along the sides of the body. Keeping the elbows straight, slowly raise the arms sideways away from the body to straight up overhead and reach for the sky turning palms in. A variation of this exercise is to begin with arms down and then raise the arms up backward, palms up as far as you are able without pain. Repeat as able up to five times.

Arm circles: Hold the arms straight out to the sides of the body with elbows locked. First, rotate the wrists in circular fashion with hand rotations, then begin to move the arms forward in small then larger circles. After one minute, reverse direction of the circles for one minute.

Arm flippers: While lying flat on your back with knees bent, extend the arms straight out to the sides and slowly raise the arms to touch in front of you. Keep the arms straight and the elbows locked. Repeat up to five times.

Elbow flexes: While sitting with hands straight down at the sides, ball the hands into fists and alternately bend the elbows and raise the fists and arms to shoulder height. Repeat for up to one full minute of exercising.

Wrist twists: Hold arms out in front with palms up and elbows touching the waist. Spread your fingers apart as far as you are able. Rotate the wrists and palms inward to palms down then rotate palms up again. Repeat as able for up to a full minute of exercise.

Wrist fan curls: While sitting, place the arms on the thighs with palms up and wrists extended over the knees. Slowly curl the hands up at the wrist. At the top of the curl, turn the palms face out and slowly push the palms down. Repeat up to five times.

Fist grips: Sitting with hands extended and arms resting on the thighs, make fists and squeeze, then relax the fist and spread and extend the fingers out as far as possible. Repeat up to five times.

Toe touches: While sitting in a chair, extend the arms and fingers straight out and, while bending at the waist, reach down toward the toes and try to touch them. (Make sure the child is seat-belted securely in the chair if necessary.) Slowly swing the extended arms upward, keeping the elbows locked, and reaching the arms straight up overhead. Repeat up to five times.

Twisters: While standing with legs slightly spread, bend the elbows and touch and hold the shoulders with the fingertips. Twist at the waist, rotating the upper torso in one direction, and then turn to the opposite direction. Do this for five movements in each direction.

Back stretches: While sitting in a chair, place the arms along each thigh with palms down on the knees. Slowly bend at the waist so the torso is bent down to the knees. Hold for a count of five and then return to the starting position. Do this up to five times.

Kick-outs 1: Sitting in a chair, grab the sides of the chair with the arms and extend one leg straight out in front of the body, lock the knee, and hold for a count of five. Alternate legs and repeat up to five times with each leg.

Kick-outs 2: Stand behind and hold onto the back of a chair. Keep the legs straight, hips still, stomach muscles tight, and do not arch your back. Stretch one leg backward behind the body keeping the heel facing the ceiling. Hold for a count of five and repeat for the other leg. Do each leg five times.

Modified sit-ups: While lying flat on the back, cross the arms on the chest, grabbing the opposite shoulders. Pull up on the head, neck and shoulders slightly to elevate the upper torso about six inches off the ground. Hold for a count of five and repeat up to five times.

Place kick: Lie flat on your back and bend the knees so the feet are also flat on the mat. Bend slightly at the waist so you can interlock the fingers under one knee. Pull the knee slightly toward the chest, then extend the leg and point the sole of the foot toward the ceiling. Hold for a count of five and repeat for the other leg. Do five times for each leg.

Scissor kicks: Lie on your side on a mat with legs straight and together. Slowly raise the top leg, keeping the leg straight, then slowly lower it to the rest position. Repeat up to five times, then reverse position and repeat for the other leg.

Froggies: Lie flat on your back on the mat. While bending the knees and spreading the knees apart, put the soles of the feet together. Spread the knees as far apart as possible without pain. Repeat up to five times.

Leg crosses: Lie flat on a mat with knees slightly bent, feet together, heels on the floor, and arms flat along the sides of the body.

Bring one knee toward the chest and hold for a count of five. Repeat for the other leg. Perform up to five timess with each leg.

Kick backs: Lie on your stomach and prop yourself up on your elbows. Bend one knee and bring it off the floor as far as possible without pain. Return to flat and repeat for the other leg. Perform up to five times for each leg.

Leg wind-ups: While sitting in a chair, cross the legs at the knees. With the top foot, pivot at the ankle, making a complete circle in the air first to the right and then to the left. Do five circles in each direction, then change legs and repeat for the other foot.

Toe paddles: Sit in a chair and remove your shoes and socks. Pull the foot and toes up toward the chest but keep the heels on the floor. Then curl the toes down toward the floor. Repeat up to five times.

ISOMETRIC EXERCISES

Head press: To help strengthen the neck muscles, place the left or right hand with palm open flat against the left or right side of the head. Using the hand to provide resistance, try to push the head to the left or right side as appropriate, alternating sides. A variation is to press the front of the head into the palm of the hand and the back of the head into interlocked fingers as well. Repeat as able up to five times.

Shoulder presses: To help strengthen the shoulder and upper back muscles, place the left hand on the right shoulder and hold firmly. Attempt to raise the shoulder against the hand pressure, holding the shoulder down. Hold for a count of five. Alternate hands and shoulders and repeat up to five times for each shoulder.

Palm presses: To help strengthen all the arm muscles, while sitting or standing, bend the elbows, pushing them straight out to the sides, and press the palms flat against each other. Hold and press for a count of five. Repeat up to five times.

Arm presses 1: To help strengthen upper arm muscles, while sitting in a chair with elbows bent, place the elbows against the back support of the chair and forcefully press the elbows backward. Hold for a count of five and repeat up to five times as able.

Arm presses 2: To strengthen the forearm muscles, while sitting, place the forearm with palm up along the thigh. Hold onto the wrist with the opposite hand and press down while trying to lift up with the first arm. Hold for a count of five. Repeat as you are able without pain up to five times for each arm.

Hand presses: To help strengthen wrist muscles, while sitting, place the left arm on the thigh palm up. Lightly press down on the palm with the other hand. Try to pull up the lower hand while holding it down with the top hand. Repeat on the other side.

Knee grabs: To help strengthen wrist and finger muscles, while sitting, place the palms of the hands on the knees and squeeze each knee with the hands for a count of five. After five, open the hands and extend the fingers as far as possible and hold for a count of five. Do this for five repetitions with each hand.

Chair twisters: To help strengthen and stretch lower back muscles, while sitting in a chair, place one hand, palm up, on the knee of the opposite leg and hold that hand with the free hand. Twist at the waist turning the upper torso and head toward the shoulder of the arm on the leg. Hold for a count of five and repeat up to five times in each direction.

Knee keepers: To help strengthen outer thigh muscles, sit on a mat with legs extended and locked straight. Place your hands on the outside of the knees and lightly press inward at the knees. Try to force the knees apart. Hold for a count of five and repeat up to five times.

Leg squeeze: To help strengthen inner thigh muscles, while sitting in a chair, place the balled fist between the knees and press the knees together. Hold for a count of five. Repeat up to five times.

Leg lifts: To strengthen rear thigh muscles, lie flat on a mat on your stomach with arms straight down along the body, palms down. Lock one leg straight and slowly raise the entire leg twelve inches. Hold for a count of five. Repeat up to five times for each leg.

Cross leg presses: To help strengthen the thigh muscles, lying flat on a mat on your back, keep your feet and ankles together, and bend the knees slightly. Raise one knee slightly toward the chest and with the hands, press against the knee to resist movement.

Hold for a count of five and repeat for the other leg. Perform up to five times for each leg.

Kick presses: To help strengthen calf muscles, while sitting in a chair, hold onto the sides of the chair, cross your legs at the ankles, placing one ankle on top of the other ankle. Use the top foot to resist movement and try to straighten out the lower leg. Hold for a count of five and reverse legs. Repeat up to five times for each leg.

Backward ankle presses: To help strengthen calf muscles, lie on your stomach while propped up on your elbows. Place one ankle over the other and use the top leg to provide minimal resistance. Try to raise the lower leg up toward the buttocks. Hold for a count of five and repeat for the other leg. Perform up to five times for each leg.

Tippy-toes: To help strengthen calf and ankle muscles, stand while holding onto the back of a chair. Stand up on the toes and hold for a count of five. Repeat up to five times. As a variation, you can move up and down on your toes up to five times.

Heel pushes: To help strengthen calf, ankle and foot muscles, sit in a chair and remove your shoes and socks. Place one foot on top of the other foot with the heel of the top foot in the toe joints of the lower foot. Try to pull up on the lower foot while gently pushing down with the upper foot. Hold for a count of five and alternate feet. Repeat up to five times with each foot.

ISOTONIC EXERCISES

Resisted shoulder shrugs: To help strengthen shoulder and upper back muscles, perform warm-up shoulder shrugs, but have someone assist by standing behind with hands lightly on the shoulders to provide minimal resistance. Hold for a count of five and repeat five times.

Resisted arm stretches: To help strengthen biceps and upper and lower back muscles, sit in a chair (securely seat-belted for safety if necessary) and extend the arms straight out toward the toes while bending at the waist. Have someone stand in front with hands on the child's hands to provide minimal resistance. Slowly raise extended arms straight up overhead. Repeat up to five times.

Resisted arm circles: To help strengthen the biceps, perform the arm circles in the warm-up section, but have someone assist by standing behind and holding the hands lightly to provide some resistance. Do five times in each direction.

Resisted arm lifts: To help strengthen the triceps, drop the arms straight down along the body. With elbows locked, slowly begin to raise the arms out sideways. Have someone standing behind to provide minimal resistance to the arms as they begin to rise. Do this for five repetitions.

Side arm presses: To help strengthen the forearm muscles, bend the right arm at the elbow along the body and ball the right fist. Using the left hand under the balled fist to resist movement, try to push down on the arm without pain. Hold for a count of five. Alternate elbows and repeat up to five times.

Chair push-ups: To help strengthen the inner forearm muscles, while sitting in a chair, firmly grasp the armrests with both hands, elbows bent out. Straighten out the arms while slightly pushing the body up. Do not push totally out of the chair. Slowly return to the sitting position. Repeat this five times.

Resisted wrist flips: To help strengthen the wrist muscles, place the right forearm on the right thigh with palm down extending over the knee. Have someone provide light and minimal resistance by placing her fingers on the back of the palm. Move the hands up at the wrists with the resistance. Repeat up to ten times for each hand.

Palm pushes: To help strengthen the wrist muscles, place one hand on the knee with the other hand across the fingers of the first hand. While pushing down with the top hand, pull up — not out — with the bottom hand. Hold for a count of five. Repeat up to five times.

Finger push-ups: To help strengthen the finger muscles, place palms together and push the fingers of each hand against the other. Push the palms out while bringing the fingers down together to the center. Slowly return to the starting position. Repeat up to five times.

Sitting leg pulls: To help strengthen the outer thigh muscles, while sitting, place the hands on the knees, palms down. Using the hands to provide minimal resistance, slowly raise one knee up a few inches toward the chest. Repeat for the other leg. Perform up to five times for each leg.

Heel walkers: To help strengthen the rear calf and ankle muscles (for individuals in wheelchairs), while sitting in a wheelchair, release the brake on the chair and raise the footrests away from the chair. Place the feet down on the ground and use the heels of the feet to pull yourself along the floor, alternating in a walking style. Continue walking along for up to twenty feet. Repeat up to five times or a total of one hundred feet.

Flying ducks: To help strengthen stomach, chest and outer thigh muscles, lying flat on the stomach, lock the arms straight and place along the body with palms up. Lift chest, head and arms up and hold for a count of five. Repeat up to five times.

Back kick lifts: To help strengthen outer thigh and calf muscles, lie on your stomach with upper torso propped up on the elbows. Cross the legs behind you at the ankle. Try to raise the lower leg by bending it at the knee while providing minimal downward pressure with the top leg. Alternate legs and repeat up to five times for each leg.

Chair curls: To help strengthen stomach and lower back muscles, while lying flat on the back, straighten the arms down along the body flat on the mat with palms flat on the mat. Slowly bend at the waist and elevate the upper torso, head and neck while bringing the arms up toward the toes. Hold for a count of five and repeat up to five times.

Backward push-ups: To help strengthen lower back, buttocks, rear thigh and rear calf muscles, lie flat on your back with arms out along the body, palms down. Bend the knees so the feet are also flat on the mat. Keeping the knees together, lift the buttocks and hips off the mat and straighten the back. Hold for a count of five and repeat up to five times.

COOLING-DOWN EXERCISES

Shoulder presses: Sit in a chair and fold the arms across the chest while holding the elbows extended out front. Move the hands back toward the shoulder and attempt to grab the shoulders. Hold for a count of five and release. Do this five times.

Arm/finger stretches: Lock the fingers together in front of the chest with elbows extended out. Slowly turn the palms down then out and push out the palms, stretching the arms straight out. Hold for a count of five and return to the rest position. Do this up to five times.

Swan dive: While standing, grab the hands behind the back and interlock the fingers. Slowly pull up and out on the hands. Keep the shoulder blades together. Stretch as far as comfortable and hold for a count of five. Repeat up to five times.

Side dives: While sitting or standing, drop arms straight down beside the body, bend down to one side and extend the fingers, trying to touch the side of the knee if you are standing and the floor if you are sitting. Do five times on each side.

Wall pushes: With back straight, stand a little more than arm's length away from a strong wall. Place the palms flat against the wall with arms parallel to the floor. Place one leg slightly ahead of the other toward the wall. Slowly bend the elbows and push in toward the wall until you feel resistance. Hold for a count of five and return to the upright position. Do this up to ten total times, alternating the inner leg.

Leg pretzels: Sit on a mat with legs out in front. Lift one leg while bending at the knee, place the leg over and on the other side of the lower leg with the foot flat on the floor and along the down knee. Hold for a count of five. Reverse positions and repeat for the other leg.

Leg flappers: Sit on a flat surface. Bend the knees and bring the feet together alongside each other. Spread the knees as far apart as possible without pain. Hold for a count of five and repeat up to five times. As a variation, you can spread the knees apart, hold the ankles and bend at the waist.

Five repetitions of an exercise is an excellent starting point for almost anyone. You have just enough movement to make a difference to the muscles and to get the sensation of how the exercise feels on the body, and you learn how to assess the exercises to see if they are appropriate for the individual both physically and emotionally. Increase the total number of repetitions by one each week to a maximum of twenty to twenty-five repetitions for each exercise. That will be sufficient for a full physical workout program for the special individual.

As stated at the beginning of the chapter, do not start anyone on an exercise regimen until you have permission from a physician. Show the physician the exercise programs you intend to introduce, and let the physician determine if any exercise is not appropriate for the child.

Of course, it isn't practical to do all of the exercises described in the chapter. There are sixty-four exercises in four areas. Choose several movements from each discipline—five would be a good starting point—and combine them into one complete exercise program for a total of twenty exercises. In total, this should take no longer than twenty minutes to complete. You may want to develop two or three different complete programs and alternate the programs on a weekly basis to help prevent boredom.

The important thing is that everyone needs exercise. The special child, whether sitting in a wheelchair or not, does not have all the opportunities to exercise that are available to the general public. These exercises can help stretch the muscles and provide oxygen to the body for energy and fitness.

Chapter Four

ADAPTABLE SPORTS

Although Special Olympics International is significantly discussed in chapter six, the sports in Special Olympics are not by any means the only sports that a challenged athlete — whether child, adolescent or adult — can participate in and enjoy. This chapter outlines many sports which are easily accessible to people with disabilities. I've included a wide range of sports — more active ones and more passive ones, sports suited to young kids and sports more appropriate for teens, group activities and individual sports, those that require a lot of mental awareness and those that don't — in an attempt to include something for every child. I've also provided some adaptive measures so the athlete can safely participate in the sport and gain from or enjoy the experience.

Many, but not all, of the devices and modifications mentioned in this chapter are sanctioned by official governing bodies of the sports. If the child you are working with is interested in tournament play, check with the sanctioning body to see if such equipment is legal in competition. The purpose of special equipment is to enable individuals to participate in sports programs of their choice. These devices are strictly assistive — not skills enhancers.

Some of the sports included in this chapter have no governing bodies and no official court sizes, so no mention is made. For more information on all of the sports, see the "Resources" section beginning on page 111.

ARCHERY

Archery is a very popular individual sport that is enjoyed in summer camp as part of a group activity and individually on private archery ranges. It is a perfect sport for competition and for individual recreational skill improvement. It is very easy to practice archery skills on a variety of ranges, outdoor and indoor. It is a year-round sport that shows no sex or age preference when it comes to skill ability or mastery. Archery can be done successfully standing up or sitting down, thus making it an excellent wheelchair sport.

Modifications to archery equipment are rather simple, and assistive devices are easily obtained. An assistive device should help the child develop archery skills and not replace the skills themselves. Two of the more necessary and popular devices are trigger releases and release cuffs. These devices help the child grasp and hold the bowstring better for the draw and exercise a smooth release.

Elbow and wrist supports stabilize the upper extremities, which in turn helps stabilize the drawn bow and arrow. They are not used as supports for equipment but rather for the individual. This is also true for standing boxes or standing supports. They allow wheelchair users to stand and be supported for a better shooting position.

When the child is totally unable to grasp or support the bow, bow supports are used to stabilize the weight of the bow and arrow. Grasping and drawing the bowstring, sighting and releasing are still up to the individual. The biggest benefit of this device is to allow recreational participation rather than competition.

The use of crossbows is a variation of archery that can be considered as another possible equipment modification to be used when the person cannot hold the bow or draw the bowstring.

Compound bows allow greater arrow accuracy with increased bow poundage. They are easier to draw and hold with stability. Mouthpieces are also used as a prosthetic device to hold and release the bowstring.

BASKETBALL

Basketball is the oldest organized sport for participation by individuals with challenges. The sport can be played with no rule adaptations or with significant rules changes, depending on the individuals playing the sport at the moment.

Ambulatory individuals play the game with virtually no rule changes. The only modification is the size of the ball to directly correlate with the size and age of the player: the smaller the person, the smaller the ball. Usually, it is the conventional five-on-five competition with full court use. Special Olympics competitions use a modified three-on-three competition on a half court, but this is to allow more teams to participate in a competition.

Wheelchair basketball players use an adapted net which allows easier return of the ball. A large square net erected around the rim funnels down to a lower rim. Below the lower rim is a ramp that collects the ball after a shot and guides the ball down a track to a ball-staging area, making it easier to collect the ball. Some leagues lower the height of the net, especially in exhibition play, or allow dribbling by bouncing the ball on the floor a few times and then carrying the ball in the lap for moving up court.

BEEP BASEBALL

Primarily used as a nonsighted participation sport, beep baseball is a derivative of baseball that allows for the same basic type of competition but with modification. This version of the game can also be played by wheelchair users and other individuals with disabilities.

According to the National Beep Baseball Association rules of 1987, there is no second base. First and third base are actually four-foot-high padded cylinders with speakers inside. The bases are placed ninety feet down their respective baselines and five feet off the foul line, which prevents a runner from colliding with a defensive player. The bases contain sounding units that buzz when activated. When the ball is hit, the base operator activates one of the bases. The runner must identify which base is activated and run to it before the ball is fielded by a defensive player. If the runner is safe, a point is scored as there is no running to other bases.

The game lasts for six innings with each team getting three outs. Each team has its own sighted pitcher and catcher. The catcher sets the target where the batter normally swings. The pitcher attempts to place the ball on the hitter's bat while pitching from twenty feet away. The pitcher calls out when the ball is tossed to alert the batter and fielders that the ball is in play. Once the ball is hit, it becomes a race between the fielders and the runner. Defensively, sighted

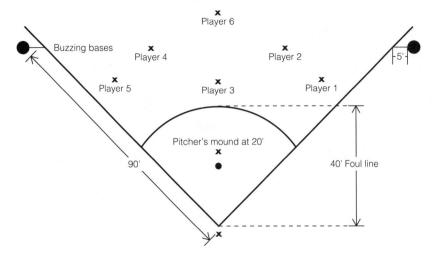

Beep baseball field dimensions and player positions.

spotters guide the players in the direction of the ball, which is also emitting an auditory signal.

Once the ball is picked up by the defense, the play is over. No throw is required. Good defensive players learn to use their bodies and the ground to trap the ball, then pick up the beeping ball and display it for the umpire's call. All players, except the pitcher and catcher while in the defensive field, must wear blindfolds at all times.

Beep baseball is best played on a large flat field free of obstructions. A baseball diamond may not necessarily be the best field to play on because of the pitching mound and differences in the grass where the base paths and field meet. The equipment needed to play the game is essentially the same as baseball with two notable exceptions: the bases, which are battery powered and emit a buzzing sound, and the ball, which is sixteen inches in diameter and emits a beep.

BOATING

Boating is such a broad and varied topic that it could fill hundreds of pages by itself. Following is a brief overview of the modifications that can make boating more accessible.

Boating encompasses a wide range of watercraft including sailboats, motorboats, and manual boats such as rowboats, kayaks and canoes. Rowing, kayaking and canoeing are all excellent means of getting physically fit. They are also good for establishing upper body strength.

Regardless of the type of vessel, the modifications are essentially the same. For boaters with upper extremity problems, adapted grips are used to hold the paddle or oar. An adapted grip may be an oversized grip, a locking grip or device such as Velcro straps to hold the hands onto the handle, or even a one-armed wing paddle for kayakers with one upper extremity.

Adapted seats support wheelchairs. The adaptations may include side and back seat supports along with seat harnesses for stability and safety. An individual may need leg and ankle stabilizers or supports to prevent tipping due to extraneous muscle movement in the lower extremities. For the vision-impaired, an auditory directional compass will help the boater keep on course.

Naturally, safety is the biggest concern when boating. All participants should be certified by the Red Cross as swimmers or at least should wear a United States Coast Guard-approved life preserver at all times.

BOCCIA

Boccia is the indoor version of Italian lawn bowling. This is an extremely exciting and competitive sport in which people of all skills and disabilities may participate. The object of the game is similar to lawn bowling. Participants attempt to get their game balls closest to a small white ball (placed near a target cross) without hitting it. Players are grouped into two teams with up to three players per team. Points are based on the total number of balls a team rolls closest to the white ball.

The court consists of two areas, the ball area and the player box area. The size of the court may vary, depending on the available area of play. Each player must stay completely within one of the six designated player boxes at all times. The game balls are soft, for easy gripping, and are slightly smaller than a baseball. Individuals with upper extremity problems can use their feet as launchers by

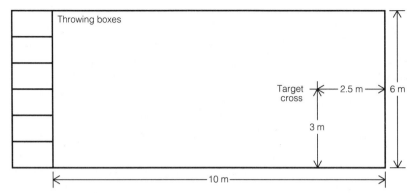

Official court dimensions for boccia.

either gripping the ball with their toes and tossing the ball or by pushing and rolling the ball down the court with the foot.

The only adaptive equipment necessary for participants with upper extremity problems is a chute or ramp down which their game balls can be launched. This ramp is totally adjustable up and down and is on a swivel base to control speed, distance and direction of the ball and can be mouth or foot activated as necessary.

BOWLING

Thousands of challenged individuals across the country and around the world are involved in the sport of bowling. Bowling is an excellent recreational as well as competitive sport. It is certainly one of this country's most popular pastimes. Modifications are minimal. Rules are essentially the same as standard bowling rules. Many challenged bowlers bowl free arm while standing up at the foul line. Wheelchair bowlers may need adaptive equipment.

Bowling balls may have a built-in, spring-loaded, retractable full-grip handle that provides an easier and more comfortable way to grip the ball. Upon release, the handle immediately retracts to flush with the surface of the ball so the ball rolls straight and true. Wheelchair bowlers may use a ring-shaped ball holder in the lap to hold the ball more easily while pushing themselves up to the foul line. Bowlers may choose to use a bowling stick if they don't have the strength to hold and roll the ball. The bowling stick is a two-pronged stick, similar to a shuffleboard stick, used to push the ball along.

Bowling ramps are the most common form of adaptive equipment. The ramps are long metal or wooden frames used to guide the ball down the alley. The athlete must decide the strength and direction of the delivery of the ball in order to knock down the pins. Most bowling lanes in the United States have at least one bowling ramp available. Most bowlers use their hands to push the ball, but others use their feet, mouth or other part of the body. Still others use a head stick or other prosthetic device to roll the ball down the ramp.

Bowling guides are the final adaptation necessary at the lanes and are used primarily for nonsighted bowlers. The guides may be metal rails down the side of the approach, a taut string tied from a weighted object at the foul line to another object in the rest area, or even a strip of carpeting down the center of the approach. The major disadvantage with the carpeting is that it must be removed for each sighted bowler and then replaced again for the nonsighted bowler.

As a training aid, many bowling alleys now have bumper bowling. Bumpers are long, inflated tubes laid in the gutters to prevent balls from entering them. They act as guides to the ball as it travels down the lane. These are highly effective in preventing frustration for the beginning bowler who needs significant encouragement. They are also highly effective when used for bowlers with mental or physical retardation.

CYCLING

Cycling is no doubt one of the country's most popular outdoor events. For many people, cycling is their major form of transportation. It is performed with equal enthusiasm around the world in developed and underdeveloped countries. Cycling is also enjoyed by a great number of physically and mentally challenged individuals.

Cycling races vary from short one- or two-hundred-meter sprints to up to ten and twenty thousand meters. Races are judged according to either a winner (first across the line) or by time trials.

Equipment adaptation can be as varied as the number of individuals in a race. Older kids can use an adult tricycle with adapted seat for support. This allows an individual with little balance or control to ride smoothly. A variation on the adult tricycle is the two-seat tricycle that allows a sighted person to be the navigator (or steer person) and power assister while a nonsighted individual is the primary means of power.

The tricycle can also be modified to be slung close to the ground with wide-set wheels for maximum stability. In addition, it can be hand powered by moving the pedal up the frame to be rotated by the hands and arms.

Prosthetic hand devices are usually not necessary other than a Velcro hand lace to hold the hand to the handlebar grip. Training for cycling is easy since there is usually an unlimited amount of roadway to navigate.

FENCING

Fencing is a traditionally European sport that does not share U.S. popularity with such sports as running, bowling and soccer. It is, however, an international sport that is recognized by many amateur athletic associations throughout the world.

Teens, but usually not younger kids, compete in the three events of foil, epee and sabre. This sport is potentially dangerous, so it is usually limited to individuals with a physical rather than a mental disability. Because of the delicate and quick movements required, competitors must be very sharp mentally. In modified competition, all competitors compete in wheelchairs.

Modifications to the rules for these events are extremely significant. The United States Fencing Association can provide complete rules and modifications.

FIELD EVENTS

Field events comprise the third largest component of competitive sports opportunities for the disabled, with swimming and track being the first two. Their popularity is due to the fact that training is easy, minimal equipment is necessary, and many competitions do not require special skills or abilities.

Field events are shot put, discus, javelin, high jump and standing long jump. In additional to these conventional events, there are several modified events that are practical, such as the distance throw, the soft discus, precision throwing, high toss, kicking and club throw. Additional variations of these events may be particular to a specific organization or governing body.

The conventional events have few or no rules modifications for any child. They are performed essentially the same as is standard. The modified events have some minimal rules modifications.

The *distance throw* is, as the name implies, an event in which the individual attempts to throw an object, usually a soft shot, as far as possible. The *soft discus* is usually a soft, round implement similar in shape and size to a conventional discus. It is thrown in the same manner and for the same effect of distance. In *precision throwing*, the person attempts to score the highest possible number of points with six throws of a bean bag at an eight-ring target placed on the ground. The *high toss* involves throwing a soft shot over a progressively higher bar, usually a pole vault bar. Competitors are given three attempts at each height with the winner the one who successfully throws the shot the highest.

There are two *kicking* events, the thrust kick and the distance kick, although both kicks are for distance. In the thrust kick, the child's foot must maintain contact with the ball at all times prior to the release. In the distance kick, the child may take a "wind-up" prior to kicking the ball.

In the *club throw*, the person must throw an Indian club for distance. All rules of the javelin toss apply in this event.

Field events are equally popular for individuals with physical and/ or mental retardation. They provide a way to test skills and compete at the same time.

FISHING

Fishing is a recreational sport to be enjoyed by all. It is included in this chapter because it has wide popularity in all walks of life with individuals of all ages. The best way to describe fishing is that it's fun! It is one of the easiest sports for individuals with challenging conditions to participate in. In addition, fishing is one of the easiest sports to adapt. Because there are no real rules to recreational fishing, there is no need to worry about rules violations.

Many commercial grasping devices are available for kids with upper extremity problems. Metal hooks that hook around the hands and arms and are then secured with a Velcro strap are one aid for holding a rod. A foam-padded hand bracket which is attached to the rod and clamps over the hand or arm is another. Persons may also use a chest harness, similar to a deep-sea waist harness, to hold and stabilize the rod. A wheelchair support pole can be attached to the arm of a wheelchair to hold the rod while an individual hooks and baits the line.

Wheelchair users are not limited in fishing. They can fish from a flat-bottom boat while in a wheelchair secured to the gunnels and transom, or they may use adapted seats for stability (see *Boating*). A United States Coast Guard-approved life preserver is recommended when out on the water. Fishing from the shore or bank is desirable by many experienced fishermen without boats.

Reels with electric winches are also available to help in reeling in the "big one," and pliers, grabbers or tongs can help remove the fish from the hook. Whatever an individual's imagination can conceive to use to help make the fishing experience more pleasurable is acceptable in fishing.

FLOOR HOCKEY

This version of hockey is a very popular sport that is easily adapted and played by children with both physical and mental retardation. The game can be played on a standard gym floor with gym mats used as boundaries. The playing area should be a minimum of twelve by twenty-four meters. Teams may have up to eleven players with five or six players at a time (depending on the organizing body) competing in the game. Players are rotated into the game in a fashion similar to ice hockey.

The games consist of three nine-minute periods. The puck is a circular felt disc with a hold in the middle. The puck can be directed around the floor by a conventional hockey stick or by a wood or fiber glass dowel or rod. The floor surface is laid out similarly to ice

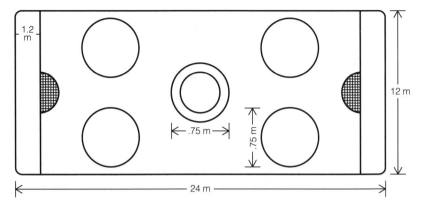

Floor hockey court dimensions.

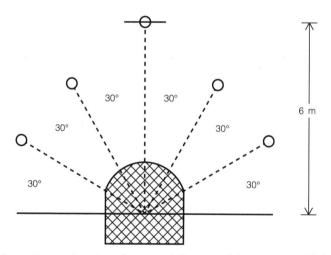

Official dimensions and settings for team skill event of shooting around the goal.

hockey with five face-off circles spaced throughout the rink and two goals, one at each end of the rink. The rules of play are similar to ice hockey.

Individuals can compete either in teams with other similarly abled athletes, or with wheelchair users while competing on all-wheelchair teams. The wheelchair version is played, however, using electric wheelchairs instead of manual wheelchairs.

Players can also compete in individual skills competitions. These skills include:

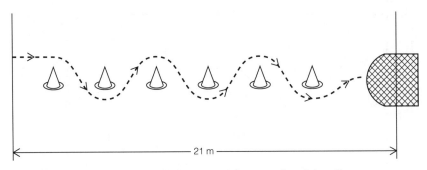

Official dimensions and settings for team skill event of stick handling.

- shooting around the goal, or shooting at the goal from a number of floor positions, with one point awarded for each goal
- passing, where points are awarded when a player successfully makes a pass between two cones placed eight meters away
- stick handling, where a player is required to maneuver the puck around a series of cones
- accuracy shooting, where a player shoots at various sections of the net for varying point accumulations
- defense, where a player is given two attempts to steal a puck from two opponents while staying between them in a confined area

All players should wear protective equipment including helmets, shin guards, elbow and shoulder pads, and goggles or a face mask.

FOOTBALL

Football is a popular and very competitive recreational sport that is easily modified whenever enough interested players gather to play a game. There are no official governing bodies of adapted football so the rules variations are more a result of custom than regulation.

There are no rules variations for deaf individuals playing the sport. The rules followed are the same as those of NCAA collegiate football or high school football. For nonsighted players, an auditory emitting football is available and the rules are loosely based on those of beep baseball.

Wheelchair users have applied the most adaptations to the game.

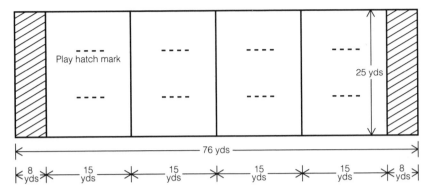

Official wheelchair football field dimensions.

While rules modifications are adjusted from league to league, here are the modifications that seem to be the most generally accepted. Teams consist of six players. Play takes place on an asphalt parking lot seventy-six yards long and twenty-five yards wide. The lot is marked off into four fifteen-yard quarters with an eight-yard deep end zone at each end of the field. The game is played in four fifteen-minute quarters with a ten-minute half time after the second quarter. Play is similar to flag or touch football and the rules loosely follow NCAA football rules. The ball is advanced either by running, where the quarterback hands off the ball, or by passing, where all players are eligible receivers. As in regular football, the object is to score touchdowns by moving the ball into the end zone.

GOAL BALL

Goal ball is a European version of team handball that was invented for blind World War II veterans. There are two teams of three players each. The game is played on a regulation gym floor and the court is divided into two sections. Goals are placed at each end of the floor. Field markings are five centimeters wide and of a distinctive texture for easy play orientation. The object of the game is to roll a ball with a bell in it across a goal line while the opposing team attempts to prevent this from happening. Teams alternate rolling the ball to either goal. The game consists of two five-minute halves with a two-minute half-time period. Two three-minute overtime periods followed by free throws are used as tie breakers.

Equipment needed is minimal. The goals are 1.3 meters high and 9 meters long. Adults use 1,500- and 2,000-gram balls, but a lighter ball should be used with kids. All players, regardless of vision, must wear a blindfold for the entire length of the game including time-out and half-time periods. Knee, elbow and hip pads are worn for protection.

GOLF

The game rules of golf are generally not modified for the challenged individual. Some acceptable variations of grips and stances are used. Other than physical limitations, there are no real restrictions, although some children may not have the necessary patience to play.

Individuals with lower extremity problems can use a chair or stool, often attached to an electric golf cart, to aid in support and stability when addressing the ball. The player must be able to walk for short distances however, because golf carts are not permitted on greens and the golfer must putt the ball on the green to hole out (get the ball in the hole).

Clubs may be lengthened or shortened as necessary to provide a correct swing plane. Shafts may be as stiff or as flexible as desired. Individuals with upper extremity problems can use a grip prosthesis to help hold the club. Many commercially available devices help in holding the club. Ask the golf professional at a local club for assistance in choosing, obtaining and using one if needed.

For blind golfers, there are no modifications to the rules other than using a sighted spotter to align the golfer to the ball and to set up the swing in the right plane.

Miniature golf is an excellent form of recreation that kids in wheelchairs can enjoy. The elements of golf remain the same without the strenuous twisting and turning necessary to strike the ball sharply.

GYMNASTICS

Gymnastics is a big part of Special Olympics International, but it is also minimally a part of other sporting organizations' roster of sports. The events are run according to high school and college level programs and rules throughout the United States. Standard events include floor exercise, parallel bars, pommel horse, rings, horizontal bar, vaulting and all-around for males. Events for females are floor exercise, balance beam, uneven parallel bars, vaulting and all-around. Women's rhythmic gymnastics include rope, hoop, ball, ribbon and all-around.

Safety is the major concern and only United States Gymnastic Federation standard equipment can be used. Using spotters is a rule variation that helps to assure safety. Emphasis is also placed on participation with success. The events are divided into four ability level groups: level A (training), level 1 (beginner), level 2 (intermediate) and level 3 (advanced). This allows many individuals to compete at their own level without frustration.

While it is true that children with physical and mental limitations may not be able to participate in all gymnastic events, many show extraordinary talent and perseverance when given the opportunity. While some events, such as the vault or balance beam, may not be appropriate for wheelchair users, these children can participate in rhythmic gymnastics, floor exercises in their chairs, or bar events if upper body strength is sufficient.

HORSEBACK RIDING

Horseback riding has long been recognized as a highly effective and therapeutic tool when working with people who are physically challenged. In addition, it is an excellent activity and sport for individuals with any disability, physical or mental.

In 1969, the North American Riding for the Handicapped Association (NARHA) was formed to introduce and regulate horseback riding for handicapped people. The goals of the organization are multifold. The organization strives to establish standards and techniques. NARHA provides manuals and other literature to members and requesting sources. It advises and accredits operating programs. In addition, the organization strives to maintain safety of the individuals through constant contact with the medical community; it makes regular inspections of operating facilities; it publishes a newsletter to keep members abreast of the changing sport; and NARHA promotes responsible research and makes it available to members.

Using special safety equipment is not only a necessity, but it also promotes a more therapeutic ride. The helmet is the first standard piece of required equipment. Only Snell Foundation-approved helmets can be used for competition, and they are recommended for recreational use also.

A body harness or waist belt helps stabilize the rider and enables assistants walking beside the horse to hold onto the rider easily. The belt or harness is a large leather device with handles on each side for the walkers.

Saddle types range from a saddle fleece to heavy-duty western saddles. The type to use depends on the physical limitation of the rider.

Riders with upper extremity difficulties can use modified reins which include a rein bar for one-handed grips. Riders can also use additional neck straps for stability.

Stirrups should be breakaway Peacock stirrups which open up when a certain amount of pressure is applied to the foot such as in a fall. Some stirrups have rubber cups attached to help keep the foot in the rig. For the above-the-knee amputee, stirrups can be raised and modified to allow for a residual limb.

Mounting blocks or platforms are the final device used to help physically challenged people get on a horse. Mounting blocks can be anything from simple wooden blocks, used to provide additional minimal height, to complete roll-up wheelchair platforms that raise the chair to horseback height and help the wheelchair user get on the horse.

ICE SKATING

Ice skating is a very popular year-round activity that can be enjoyed by children with disabilities. In spite of its long presence in the world, the therapeutic value of ice skating has only recently been noted and accepted. It significantly benefits people with lower extremity difficulties and even lower limb amputations.

Competitive ice skating comprises the sports of speed skating and figure skating. The rules modifications for both sports are minimal, primarily focusing on placing athletes in competition divisions.

Speed skating events include the 100, 300, 500, 800 and 1,000 meter distances as well as a 10-meter skate race, a 10-meter assisted race and a 30-meter slalom race.

Figure skating events include single, pairs and ice dancing along with five individual skills contests.

Adaptive equipment includes the popular skate walker to aid in stability for individuals with lower limb impairments. This device resembles a regular walker but has a pyramidal design with an extra-wide bottom with runners attached. Skaters may use an outrigger, a pole or crutch with a skate blade attached, to aid in stability. Ankle and foot mafo supports (hard plastic shells) are used for additional lower limb stability. Even wheelchairs can be adapted to slide on the ice by using a modified pair of snowmobile steering skis strapped to the wheels. A skating partner pushes the wheelchair along. Although noncompetitive, wheelchair skating is an excellent recreational sport.

ICE SLEDDING

Ice sledding is a very popular sport in Canada. It is basically ice skating while sitting down. This is a new sport for challenged individuals and rules and regulations are pretty much left up to the individuals who sponsor events. The sport is both recreational and competitive. Speed events are generally raced at the same distances as ice skating events.

The primary equipment is the ice sled or *sledge*. Many skaters use a stripped down and shortened wheelchair frame attached to long steel runners for speed. The individuals propel themselves using two picks, which are essentially shortened ski poles, one in each hand. In Canada, the events are held on large frozen ponds to minimize turning and the need to brake quickly. However, indoor ice rinks offer an acceptable alternative.

LAWN BOWLING

Lawn bowling is a highly competitive and recreational sport popular throughout Europe; it is also enjoying a resurgence here in the United States. The game is played on a regulation lawn bowling court. Unlike boccia, which uses bowling rams or chutes, there are no rules modifications. Scoring is the same as in regulation lawn bowling.

Because of the lack of rules modification, this sport can be limiting to some individuals, especially for those who have upper extremity problems. But the balls can be rolled using either the arms or the legs and feet, and so it can be enjoyed by individuals with a variety of challenging conditions.

MOTOR SOCCER

This unique adaptation of the game of soccer is played primarily by individuals who are severely disabled and in motorized wheelchairs, although anyone in a motorized wheelchair can engage in the sport. The game is played on a regulation basketball court with a three-meter goal line marked on each end. Court size and surface can be changed to suite availability. The game is played in two thirty-minute halves with a ten-minute half-time period. The primary object is to push the ball over the opponent's goal line.

Two major concerns are safety for the individual's lower extremities and selection of a game ball. A squared-off bumper box, fitted into the footrests of the wheelchair where the rubber tips are usually placed, is used as both a ball pusher and a leg and foot protection device. The ball used must be large enough that it can't squeeze under the bumpers of any of the wheelchairs in play, and it must be soft enough to provide adequate protection if it should bounce up and hit a competitor in the face. Trial and error using various types of balls is suggested.

QUAD RUGBY

Quad rugby is a conglomeration of several sports, taking the finer or more exciting aspects of basketball, soccer and hockey and combining them into one strange and unique activity. It is played primarily by quadriplegics who are often left out of the excitement of faster team sports. The game is played on a basketball court defined by pylons and is played with a volleyball. The playing time consists of two twenty-minute halves. The object of the game is to get the ball across the opponent's goal line, which is eight meters wide, using passing throwing, batting, rolling, dribbling or carrying—in essence, by any means possible.

Equipment modification is almost nonexistent. Using regular wheelchairs is encouraged and an official volleyball is all that is required. Some players may use gloves for better ball control and to prevent minor injuries such as callouses or finger sprains.

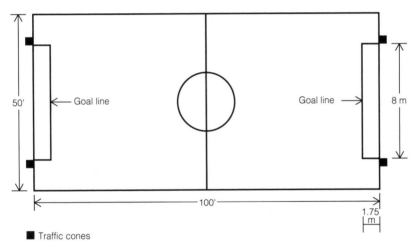

50'

Goal line

Goal line

8 m

100'

1.75 m

■ Traffic cones

Official quad rugby court dimensions.

RACQUETBALL

Wheelchair racquetball is unique in that it is the only sport specific to individuals in wheelchairs that has been adopted by its nonchallenged governing body (the United States Racquetball Association) as an official division. The rules changes and modifications are minimal and court dimensions are exactly the same. Standard racquets and balls are used by the wheelchair participants. Most participants choose to use the fast, light competition-style wheelchair. The only type of chair banned is the kind with black tires that can mar the surface of the court. Players with upper extremity difficulties may choose to use grip enhancers or supports to hold the racquet more easily.

ROLLER SKATING

Roller skating is such a popular sport in North America that it has been included in the Pan American Games and the U.S. Olympic Festival. Roller skating can be enjoyed by participants who have almost any physical or mental disability.

Competitive speed races, dance and artistic style events may be participated in. The latter two adhere to the basic rules and figures of ice skating.

Adaptive equipment is primarily the skate walker, which is similar to the one also used in ice skating, but modified to replace the blade runners with wheels. Some children may require a lower extremity support to help in foot, leg and ankle support. For the visually impaired, use of a tether or sighted guide is suggested.

Races are run on an official 100-meter nonbanked oval track, while artistic events are held on any suitable and obstruction-free gym-type floor. No other special equipment or rules modifications are necessary.

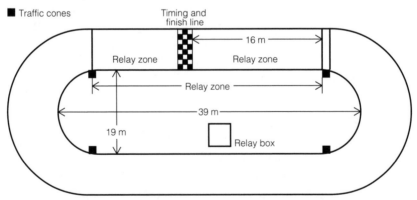

Official roller skating track dimensions for speed skating. This is a 100 meter track.

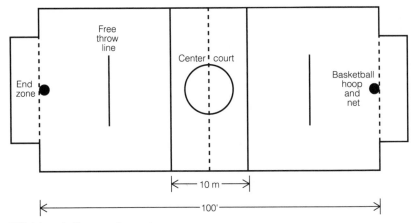

Official rugball court dimensions.

RUGBALL

Rugball is an excellent sport for any person with minimal catching and throwing skills. Rugball distinguishes itself by eliminating player mobility while in possession of the ball. This helps enforce the primary goals of the game — teamwork and cooperation. Each player on the team must contribute for the team to be successful. If a player does not have minimal catching and throwing skills, rules modifications are permitted to allow these individuals to play.

The team consists of five players per side. The game is played on a regulation basketball court. The only equipment is a standard volleyball or a soft Nerf-like ball to aid in gripping. All players, including the nonchallenged, are required to be in wheelchairs during play unless all players are ambulatory.

The game is played in two twenty-five-minute halves with a five-minute half-time period. Each half starts with a kickoff. Once the ball is in play, the player with the ball must stop and may only pivot his wheelchair. The ball possessor must pass the ball within five seconds or lose possession of the ball.

Scoring is as follows: Four points, or a "try," are scored when a player catches the ball in the end zone or pivots across the end line while in possession of the ball. A two-point conversion can be attempted after a "try" is scored. Conversions are free throws to a basketball basket from the standard foul line.

SHOWDOWN

Showdown is a competitive sport which is a cross between air hockey and table tennis. It is played primarily in Canada and Europe but it is rapidly growing as a sport for the visually impaired throughout North America.

The object of the game is to score eleven points by making goals or by other means. The game is played on a twelve-foot-long by four-foot-wide table which stands thirty-five inches above the floor. The table is completely enclosed by an eight-inch-high wall, and has a fifteen-inch-high center screen mounted on top of the side boards. The center screen divides the table in two yet allows the ball to pass freely underneath. The screen also prevents players who have some vision from seeing the actions of their opponents. Sunken goals are built in at each end of the table.

The game is played with a fifteen-inch-long, three-and-one-half-inch-wide handled paddle called a bat. The ball is a twenty-gram plastic ball, 2.75 inches in diameter, into which five to seven BBs are placed to provide noise and to decrease bouncing.

Scoring is as follows: two points for a goal scored; two points for the opponent if a player hits the ball into the screen; one point for the opponent if the player hits the ball off the table; and one point for the opponent if a player touches the ball with any part of the body other than the wrist. The player who is first to reach eleven points with at least a two-point lead is the winner.

SKIING

Skiing is no doubt one of the most popular recreational and competitive sports in the world today. Its growing popularity in the challenged world is attributed to its easy modifications and its therapeutic qualities.

To enable kids with any type of challenge or handicapping condition to ski, there are five primary types of skiing systems: the buddy system used by deaf and blind skiers and by those with mental retardation; three-track skiing used by amputees, post-polio, traumatic and hemiplegic skiers; four-track skiing used by skiers with mental retardation and those with cerebral palsy, muscular dystrophy and multiple sclerosis; the ski bra used in four-track skiing by those with muscular dystrophy, spina bifida, paraplegia and cerebral palsy; and sit skiing used primarily by those with paraplegia and others who cannot use their legs for support.

The *buddy system* involves using a second, usually sighted, skier or nonchallenged guide to aid the challenged skier down the hill or trail. The system is basically a fifty-fifty proposition, with each party sharing the responsibility of the skiing equally, although the guide does assume a bigger responsibility for the safety of both skiers.

Three-track skiing is the largest category of assisted skiing. It involves using one center ski and two outrigger skis held in the hands to provide stability, support and steering ability. The outriggers are worn like crutches but with small skis attached to the ends. They are height adjustable and the bottom runner ski will only allow up to thirty degrees of flexibility. A cord attached to the runner flips the runner up out of the way when pulled and the remaining pole can be used as a crutch. Three-track skiers are usually single-leg amputees or individuals who can support themselves on one but not both legs.

Four-track skiing is like three-track skiing except that the skier uses two skis instead of one ski to provide additional support and stability.

A *ski bra* is a short, strong metal bar that is attached to the tips of both skis of a pair to prevent them from crossing each other. The ski bra is primarily used when skiing with poles but is also used extensively by four-track skiers.

Sit skiing is, as its name implies, downhill skiing while sitting in a highly adapted ski sled. The sit ski is used most by those individuals with lower extremity impairments. Each sled is adapted to the requirements of the individual. Modifications include back and side supports, roll bars, safety straps and tethers. In addition, the bottom of the sled is adapted either for speed, by being fitted with a single ski, or for stability, with no ski.

For propelling and stability, skiers may use shortened poles, ice picks, kayak-style paddles, or even a hand-knuckle protection glove.

A long tether allows a sit skier to travel downhill while a qualified rear skier holds onto it. This prevents the sit skier from going too fast or in the wrong direction. Sit skiers who have demonstrated compliance and competence while using the sit ski may be untethered to ski freely.

Finally, individuals with just upper extremity problems can use an adapted-grip ski pole to allow for better gripping, greater stability and more streamlined aerodynamics so the poles don't drag when going downhill.

SLALOM

Slalom is short-track racing through an obstacle course performed primarily by wheelchair athletes. Slalom requires speed and agility with the chair, but it can be enjoyed by wheelchair users with almost any type disability and any type wheelchair, motorized or not. Competitors are classified according to type of wheelchair used, age and body strength.

Two common courses usually are laid down in slalom: a short track thirty-four meters long and a long track fifty-nine meters long. Obstacles include a figure-eight pylon negotiation, ramps, and an area where the participant must maneuver the chair forward and backward. Penalty time is awarded for minor infractions and added to the competitor's total time. Failure to complete the course or to navigate the course in the prescribed manner results in disqualification.

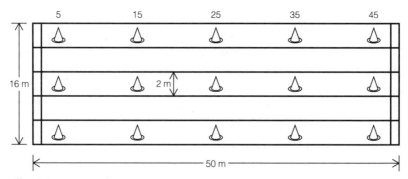

Official dimensions for a 50 meter slalom course.

SLEDGE HOCKEY

Invented in Canada, sledge hockey provides an alternative to ice hockey. It certainly encompasses the thrill, speed, power, and even danger of ice hockey, but in a manner adapted for challenged individuals.

The game is played in accordance with International Ice Federation hockey rules with only minor changes on a regulation ice rink. Each team consists of six members using a rubber puck. Helmets, face masks, gloves and elbow pads are required.

The primary and most unusual piece of equipment is the ice sledge. It is an oval metal frame with three points of contact to the ice—two skate-like blades and a small runner. Attached seats and backrest are adjusted in height and width according to the player. Leg straps hold the legs in place to provide greater stability and safety.

The players use "picks," or shortened hockey sticks with the blades cut off, to propel themselves across the ice and to shoot and control the puck. Each pick has serrated edges at the end of the shaft for better control. Some players use Velcro strips to help hold the stick in the heavy and sometimes awkward hockey glove.

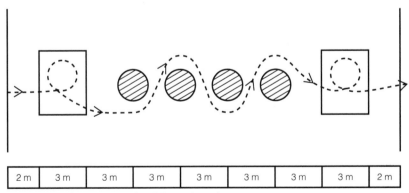

2 m	3 m	3 m	3 m	3 m	3 m	3 m	3 m	2 m

Official dimensions for a wheelchair obstacle course.

SOCCER

Although soccer has not gained the popularity in the U.S. that it has throughout the rest of the world, it remains a fun and competitive sport. Minimal equipment is required so it is an ideal sport for challenged individuals. Almost any individual, regardless of type and degree of disability, can participate in the sport.

Adaptations necessary for the game include a shortened field and smaller nets. The game is played on an eighty-by-sixty-meter field. The goals are reduced in size to two meters in height and five meters in width. Teams consist of either six or seven players on the field (depending on the local governing body). Players compete in age groups.

Many leagues hold individual skills competitions in addition to games. These include dribbling, passing, throw-ins and shooting or kicking events. Teams can participate in similar team skill events.

Amputees can also enjoy soccer with few modifications to the rules. The players run around the field on crutches and strike at the ball with the remaining limb. If there is a shortage of eligible players, non-amputees may play on crutches but one leg must be immobilized for game purposes.

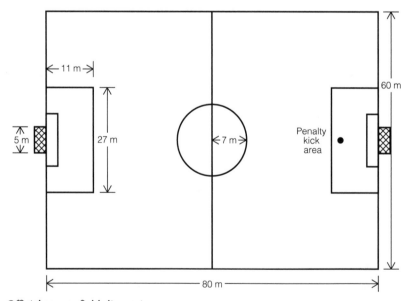

Official soccer field dimensions.

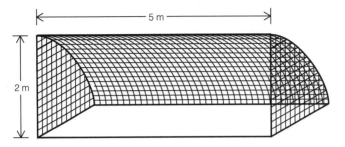

Official dimensions for a soccer goal.

While there is no sanctioned league for sight-impaired individuals, the sport is easily modified for their benefit as well. Play can be conducted with brightly colored balls or a beep-style ball. Using brightly colored flags, cones and rope to mark the sidelines is recommended. An audible goal locator can be used as in beep baseball and the goal posts are painted with bright colors for better visibility. This sport is nearly impossible for totally blind individuals to play, but they should be given every opportunity to attempt to play the sport.

SOFTBALL

Take a stroll through the playgrounds of the United States on almost any day of the year and somewhere you will see players playing this most popular team sport. This is a sport that can be enjoyed by kids of any size, any athletic ability, and any physical or mental challenge.

In Special Olympics, the sport is played with minimal rules modifications and in either regulation fashion or individual and team skills competitions. Two variations of the team events include slow-pitch and tee ball. Individual events include base race, hitting for distance and throwing. International Softball Federation rules are used in all events.

Individuals in wheelchairs can also participate in this sport, but must be in wheelchairs with footrests. The modifications for wheelchairs include a wider first base (thirty inches) with four-foot-diameter base circles for easier turns and a pitcher's box instead of a

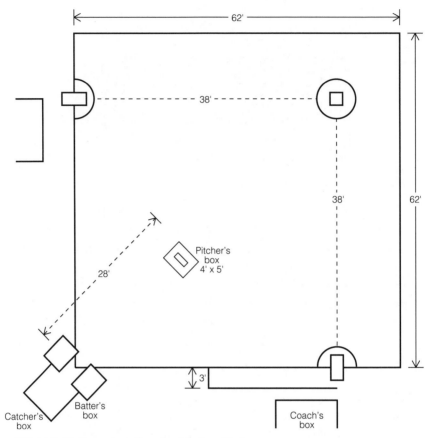

Official field dimensions for wheelchair softball.

pitcher's mound and pitching rubber. The infield is shortened to fifty feet long with thirty-eight-foot-long base paths. Play takes place on a hard blacktop surface rather than a grassy field.

SWIMMING

Swimming is one of the most popular and therapeutic activities enjoyed by people with physical disabilities. In fact, it is considered to be the *most* therapeutic recreational activity that a challenged individual can participate in. It is also one of the top three participatory sports for the challenged person. One major problem with the sport, however, is finding an accessible and supervised pool. Most therapeutic pools are in such constant use by organized programs that there is little opportunity for recreational use, and pools that are open to the general public are not appropriate for individuals with limitations.

In addition to the lack of accessibility of a pool, another major drawback is the lack of aquatic staff trained not just for general aquatics but for challenged-adapted aquatics. To be considered an adapted therapeutic pool, a pool should have portable lifts to raise and lower a swimmer into the water, access stairs from a wheelchair to the water, and an access ramp down into the pool.

Swimmers, if amputees, may choose to use some adaptive equipment to better help themselves in the pool, or they may choose to swim without adaptive devices. There is no evidence that swimming with a device is any more or less beneficial than without. Swimmers with upper extremity amputations usually choose to use prosthetic paddles or arm extenders to produce upper limbs of equal length.

Blind or visually impaired swimmers usually have little or no need for rules or equipment modification. Some pools may use a beeper device as a guide for the swimmers. Other swimmers may choose to use a "tap stick" which their coach strikes against the water surface or side wall when it is time for a turn. In other cases, especially for the backstroke, the guide flags are lowered close to the water for easier sighting.

Personal flotation devices are generally not used in adaptive aquatics except for beginning swimmers with severe to profound mental and physical retardation. Beginning swimmers tend to rely too much on the device and not enough on their own bodies for movement and flotation. They also gain a false sense of security and resist attempts to move away from using the device. Swimmers' dependence on floats should decrease as they gain better control and mastery of a stroke or gain more confidence in the water.

In any event, flotation devices are used since most aquatic events are not held as competitive events anyway. When events are held competitively, challenged swimmers swim the same strokes and distances as nonchallenged swimmers, so few rules modifications are necessary.

Diving events are usually not held competitively except by Special

Olympics and The American Athletic Association for the Deaf. You can consult rules specific to these organizations for individuals interested in diving.

TABLE TENNIS

Table tennis requires very few rules modifications and equipment adaptations to be enjoyed by challenged individuals. In competition, the games are played in accordance with the United States Table Tennis Association rules with modifications only specific to delivery of the ball. The participants are grouped mainly by age class and playing ability rather than by disability.

In sanctioned competition, tables cannot be modified. In non-sanctioned play, tables can be height-adjustable to match the competitors. A table may have side walls or rails to help keep the ball on the table. For the visually impaired, the surface of the table may be painted white and the ball painted orange for better visibility.

Paddles may be modified in both sanctioned competition and nonsanctioned play. The paddles may have alternative grips or grip straps to help hold the paddle. A player with no grip can use a cuff attached to the wrist to hold the paddle. Free-swinging arm supports in which the upper extremity rests can be attached to wheelchair arm rests help provide stability to the arms for individuals with upper extremity problems.

Table tennis can be enjoyed by individuals of any age and with any physical or mental disability.

TEAM HANDBALL

Team handball is a competitive and recreational sport that offers the challenged person the opportunity to develop and practice catching, throwing and running to enhance team-playing skills. Team handball is a fast-paced, noncontact sport that combines the basic elements of several sports and serves as an excellent training game to help develop these additional sports in the future.

The game is played on a court slightly larger than a basketball court with seven players — six active, or court, players and a goalie. The six court players play both offense and defense. The object of

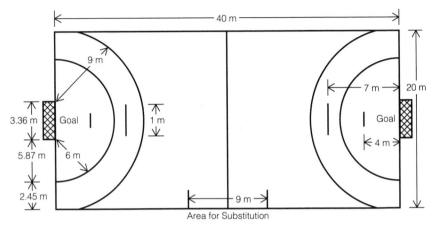

Official court dimensions for team handball.

the game is simple: Move the ball up court and attempt to throw the ball past the goalie for a score. Games consist of two thirty-minute halves with no time-outs. Player substitutions are permitted during the game.

The game is easily adapted for both the physically challenged and the mentally challenged. For players with mental retardation, modifications include a decreased court size, decreased number of players, decreased length of game, and the use of a heavy foam ball. The ball reduces the chance of body contact among players. Mentally challenged individuals may also participate in league-sanctioned individual skill events at their own level.

The game is also slightly modified to accommodate wheelchair users. There are nine players to a side, seven court players and two goalies, and they play on a basketball court. The players who control the ball are only allowed three seconds in which they must decide what to do with the ball. The court markings are similar to team handball except that there is a goalies' area in which only the goalies may play. All players, regardless of skill level, follow FIH (Federation Internationale de Handball) rules.

The only equipment needed is a ball and two goals. For ambulatory players, the ball is usually a hard leather-covered ball about the size of a cantaloupe. The ball can vary in size and weight according to the age, ability and sex of players. Wheelchair players use a soft ten-inch playground ball. Mentally challenged players use a hardened foam ball. The goals measure two meters high by three meters wide.

TENNIS

Tennis is one of the fastest-growing sports for individuals with a physical or mental challenge in the United States today. There are minimal adaptations in rules or equipment, high availability of facilities and low costs. The United States Tennis Association (USTA) is striving to accommodate the challenged person with a set rules base.

In wheelchair tennis, the most significant rules change is the "two-bounce" rule in which a ball must be returned after no more than two bounces. The only equipment modification that may be necessary is a gripping device for the racket. Depending on the severity of a player's upper extremity problem, the solution may be something as simple as a hand wrap to keep the hand around the racket grip, or it may be as complicated as full grip replacement with wrist cuff and wrist supports.

For players with mental retardation, tennis is enjoyed exactly as in the USTA rules and employs the two-bounce rule. Special Olympics participants can compete in singles, doubles or mixed doubles events, and they can take part in individual skills competitions including target serve, target bounce, racket bounce and return shot.

Players with other challenges can also play tennis but with no rules modifications at all. No allowances are made to accommodate, for example, blind or deaf players.

TOSS DARTS

Developed by Eric Dressler at Woods Services in Langhorne, Pennsylvania, in 1991, toss darts is quickly becoming a highly competitive and enjoyable recreational sport for individuals with severe to profound mental and physical retardation.

Similar to lawn darts played outdoors, this sport can be played either outdoors on the grass or a parking lot, or indoors in a gym or even a classroom. The game court consists of an eight-foot-diameter circle with increasingly one-foot-smaller concentric circles inside the outer circle, similar to an archery bullseye target, laid out on the floor. It can be painted permanently on the surface or temporarily laid out with fluorescent tape or connecting circle rings. Each circle and even portions of circles are allotted points with the highest points closest to the center.

The child tosses six round-headed, weighted indoor lawn darts one at a time at the circle from anywhere from three to ten feet away, depending on ability. One dart painted a different color is worth double value. Points are accumulated over three trials.

There are no rules modifications necessary for ambulatory players over wheelchair athletes or for less severely impaired individuals over the more severely impaired. The only recommended modification is to group competitors by severity and type of disability.

TRACK

Track events are the most popular Special Olympics events for challenged athletes competing in a single event, based on number of participants and number of events.

Rules are in accordance with The Athletic Congress of the USA (TAC) and the International Amateur Athletic Federation (IAAF) for all participants with minor modifications for specific disabilities.

Fifty percent of participants are in wheelchairs. The wheelchairs used by serious athletes include those with significant modifications in terms of weight and streamline ability and maneuverability. A person with a regular chair can participate equally. Runners using crutches also participate in track events in separate classes and heats. Currently, all participants using crutches, canes or walkers compete in one class category.

Visually impaired runners can also compete. For short distances, runners may be aided by a caller system. Runners compete individually against the clock down a single lane with a caller at the finish line calling out the lane number for the runner. If the runner begins to veer off course, the number is changed to indicate that the runner is running off course, so the runner can make adjustments. For longer distances, sighted partners run with and are tethered to the runners with fifty-centimeter ropes. A sighted partner is not permitted to run ahead of a blind partner, but the pair is allotted two lanes to run in. As the tether tightens or slackens, the blind runner is alerted that they are running off course and can adjust accordingly.

Runners can also compete using prosthetic devices, not to aid in the skills of running, but for foot, ankle or lower extremity support.

Special Olympics offers thirty-eight sanctioned events including a ten-meter assisted walk, a twenty-five-meter walk and ten-meter wheelchair dashes. Competitors are grouped according to ability, and qualifying heats are held to assure competitiveness. Participants are placed in heats according to age, sex and ability.

VOLLEYBALL

Volleyball is both a competitive and recreational sport that can be enjoyed by those of nearly any physical or mental challenge. Modifications to the game are very minimal, with smaller court size and lower net height as the only rules modifications. Many challenged athletes, however, choose to play the sport with regulation net height and court sizes.

For players with upper and lower extremity problems, two versions of the game are played, depending on which limb is affected. For those with upper limb problems, a standing version of the game is played with prosthesis devices on. For those with lower limb problems, there is sit volleyball. The sitting version of the game is played with six players per team on a smaller court with a lower net. This version allows children with spinal injuries, polio, and other lower extremity problems to play. Generally, all standard rules apply.

For the hearing impaired, a red flag can be used instead of a white flag as a signalling device. For visually impaired players, an audio emitting signal ball may be used.

Those with mental retardation participate in team events using a lowered net, a lighter ball, and a serving line which has been moved forward. A time limit of thirty minutes of play may also be applied.

Special Olympics volleyball events include volleyball juggle, volleyball pass, volleyball toss and hit for those with more severe disabilities. Individuals may also compete in individual skills events such as volleying, serving, forearm passing, hand passing and spiking.

WRESTLING

Wrestling may be the one pure sport in which the challenged participant can compete with few or no rules modifications. Competition is usually in freestyle wrestling; however, Greco-Roman wrestling (which does not allow offensive leg maneuvers) is also offered. Rules for visually impaired and hearing impaired wrestlers are identical to standard rules with the exception of a finger touch to start for blind competitors. Wrestling is prohibited in Special Olympics due to risk of injury to athletes.

A number of sports, athletic events and activities have been described here. Most certainly, the number is overwhelming. Keep in mind though, that this list is not comprehensive; many, many other sports out there are being modified daily for greater participation.

Not every athlete will want to compete in all or even most of the sports. The large number of sports included here is to inspire all children, regardless of physical or mental ability, and to provide a challenge to compete to all children.

One final note. It is imperative, in my opinion, that above and beyond anything an athlete does, it is important to *have fun*! Don't let the competition of the sport outweigh the enjoyment. We all take part in a sport for enjoyment. When it stops being fun, we usually quit the sport. Don't push the special child into something that he or she may not want to be a part of. Do not make him or her an extension of yourself and of your feelings, ideals and aspirations. Let him or her make the decision to compete and participate. Above all, *have fun*!

Chapter Five

INTEGRATION AND MAINSTREAMING

MAINSTREAMING

In April 1976 the Delegate Assembly of the Council for Exceptional Children, the major professional organization of special educators, adopted the following statement on mainstreaming:

Mainstreaming is a belief which involves an educational placement procedure and process for exceptional children, based on the conviction that each such child should be educated in the least restrictive environment in which his educational and related needs can be satisfactorily provided. This concept recognizes that exceptional children have a wide range of special educational needs, varying greatly in intensity and duration; that there is a recognized continuum of educational settings which may, at any given time, be appropriate for an individual child's needs; that to the maximum extent appropriate, exceptional children should be educated with nonexceptional children; and that special classes, separate schooling, or other removal of an exceptional child from education with nonexceptional children should occur only when the intensity of the child's special education and related needs is such that they cannot be satisfied in an environment including nonexceptional children, even with the provision of supplementary aids and services.

While providing a philosophical framework, this statement of the Council for Exceptional Children is more of a conceptual rather than a practical and operational definition. A much more specific definition of mainstreaming has evolved out of a major federal project on the efforts of mainstreaming referred to as Project PRIME

(Programmed Re-entry Into Mainstream Education). The research team of Kaufman, Gotlieb, Agard and Kulic, in an article emanating from Project PRIME, states:

... *mainstreaming refers to the temporal, instructional, and social integration of eligible exceptional children with normal peers based on an ongoing, individually determined, educational planning and programming process and requires clarification of responsibility among regular and special education administrative, instructional, and support personnel.*

According to this definition, there are three components to mainstreaming:

1. Integration
2. Educational planning and programming
3. Clarification of responsibilities

It is important to examine each aspect of mainstreaming to see how it fits in with the educational-sports models that are advocated in this book. It is also helpful to examine two models for mainstreaming and to examine the problems associated with mainstreaming.

Mainstreaming Models

Two disciplines advocate two different types of mainstream integration: the *zero reject* model and the *fail-save* model. In the zero reject model, the child is placed entirely in the nonspecial environment. The teachers, coaches and volunteers are trained on behalf of the child in direct regard to the child's needs and benefits. The child becomes a part of the "team" as a full-fledged member with no turning back. In this method, children may feel overwhelmed at the idea of total integration. They may feel that they are being abandoned and are without recourse if they become frustrated. Some children will be frightened and apprehensive.

In the fail-save model, the child is gradually integrated into the nonspecial environment. A resource teacher or facilitator acts as a transition person to gradually train the staff involved on behalf of the child. The child may only participate in an activity on a limited basis to start, with each successive session made longer and, consequently, more comfortable for the child. As needs arise, the staff is trained in how to handle a particular situation. In this approach, the child may become confused about his or her role in the activity: Am I or am I not a member of the team? Why am I only attending certain practices on select days?

Neither of the two models offers any real advantage or disadvantage over the other. Both have their strong points and their weak points. It is really up to the child and the parent together with the activity directors and organizers to decide which system they feel would work best for the child.

Considerations for Mainstreaming

The decision to mainstream a special child must be based on the organization's ability to provide instruction that will benefit the child in a regular athletic or educational program; it is not necessarily based on the severity of the disability.

When the parent and the professional support staff evaluate whether and in what areas to mainstream a special needs child, several considerations need to be examined. These considerations are:

- the child's desire to be mainstreamed
- the child's current skill levels in the area or sport under consideration
- the minimum skills needed to benefit from instruction in the regular setting
- the kind of instructional program and approaches to which the child responds best
- the organizational structure and the demands of the mainstream program
- the total number of other children in the program
- the presence of other special needs children in the program (it is often desirable to have more than one special needs child in the program at one time)
- the attitude of the mainstream coach, volunteer or instructor

toward working with children with special needs

- the mainstream coach's skill, experience and degree of success in working with children with similar disabilities
- the availability to the mainstream coach of any special materials and support equipment needed to work with the child
- the support available to the mainstream coach from other mainstream coaches and teams
- the likelihood that the special needs child will be accepted and supported by peers and teammates and the opportunities for positive social interaction
- the athletic and emotional support the special needs family is able to give the special needs child to reinforce the efforts of the mainstream coach

INTEGRATION

It is the opinion of many that temporal integration, that is, placing the exceptional child in the regular classroom or social setting for a specific length of time during the day, is just not sufficient. In addition, a mandated social and instructional integration program should be established and followed with nonspecial peers. In fact, instructional integration (the classroom) along with social integration (sports) are probably the most critical elements of mainstreaming.

The special child's instruction, both in the classroom and on the playing field, should be designed to encourage participation in activities with nonspecial children, as long as the task is not too difficult. This is not easily accomplished and no doubt keeps many mainstreaming efforts from succeeding. The question arises as to what is too difficult and what is too easy or not challenging enough. There is a delicate balance between the two that can be tipped by even the slightest miscalculation. Many times it will be left up to the child to determine present levels when it should be a team decision — the team being the child, the parent, the educators, and other care professionals involved in the child's programming.

Also, the percent of the school day that is taken up in the classroom—both mainstreamed and special—must be balanced against the time for social integration on the playing field. It has been found that when a child is integrated for either a larger (about 90) percent or smaller (about 30) percent of the time, the child does better than when mainstreamed for just about half the day. The child is better accepted by his or her peers in the upper and lower percent cases.

EDUCATIONAL PLANNING AND PROGRAMMING

The educational and social programs of the mainstreamed child need to be planned carefully. Simply placing him or her in a regular classroom or sports setting with the regular curricular goals of the class or the normal activities and exercises of the team is not enough and can in fact be harmful both physically and emotionally. Special effort must be made to plan and program for the unique needs of each special child so each can derive the maximum benefits from participating in the regular classroom and on the field. For this to occur, supportive personnel and services—parents, teachers, coaches, physical therapy, speech therapy, occupational therapy— should be available for both the child and the regular classroom teacher and regular team coach.

CLARIFICATION OF RESPONSIBILITIES

Although in some mainstreaming situations the regular teacher or coach must assume total responsibility for the special child, ideally, additional special education personnel will be involved. Most often, this will be a resource person.

When both special and regular personnel are working with the special child, there may be confusion as to who is responsible for what. It is important to delineate these roles carefully and clearly so the child's total needs can be met. It is not important who does what. What is important is that all responsibilities be covered. No area should be a "gray" area and no team member should be less than specific as to their coverage. The mainstream team members should decide themselves the areas of responsibility they feel most comfortable with. This way no team member should feel that a job has been thrust upon them which they are not ready to accept.

PROBLEMS WITH INTEGRATION AND MAINSTREAMING

As should be obvious by now, mainstreaming is not always easily implemented. The definition of mainstreaming states how it should be carried out in order for it to work. Mainstreaming is still too new a concept to have been submitted to significant and long-term research, thus its efficiency is not fully known. However, it should be noted that many trained support service personnel are warning that mainstreaming cannot be viewed as a cure-all.

Originally there were fears that it may be just another passing educational or social fad, but fortunately those fears have been proved wrong. To prevent mainstreaming from going the way of other educational fads, it is important that it be used properly, keeping the special needs child in mind at all times, and that it not be done just for the sake of mainstreaming. The idealistic goals of mainstreaming must be kept distinctly separate from its execution to avoid placing unrealistic expectations on the children. However, if there are some failures, the concept of mainstreaming should not be abandoned simply because it may not have been implemented properly. The fact remains that even with years of experience behind the implementors, mainstreaming is an extremely difficult concept to put into place.

Once the decision to mainstream a child into the regular classroom or sporting event has been made, the appropriate method of service has been chosen, the professional volunteer staff have been educated, and the adaptive equipment and rules have been ordered and modified, there are still some possible barriers the special child must hurdle to benefit most effectively from mainstreaming. The first consideration is the child's peers and their families and the actions, reactions and emotions that they—both the special child and nonspecial peers—will encounter. The second is the child's own emotional and spiritual strength.

Resistance of Facilitators

One of the biggest problems with the mainstreaming movement is the assumption that it can and will be readily accepted by the general population who are required to carry out the principles of mainstreaming. The weak link in the chain is the regular classroom educator and weaker still is the nonprofessional coach, trainer or volunteer on a nonspecial team who is required to accept mainstreaming and its principles. Some mainstream teams and classrooms have been quickly established with little planning and thought. Many questions remain as to how to prepare general educators, the child's peers, and the coaches and volunteers who run the teams. Until the mid-1970s, college students in general education had little exposure to special education courses. Many coaches and volunteers have little or no higher education directed toward special children and little direct exposure to the special child. Their problem is even greater and more challenging.

The fact that the regular education, sports coaching system and general population are not ready to deal with physically and mentally challenged children is evident. A survey of professional educators and care workers showed that only 88 percent of those interviewed indicated that they even knew about the characteristics and social integration of challenged individuals. Of that 88 percent, only 27 percent said they felt comfortable and qualified to offer services to those individuals. For mainstreaming to be an accepted, efficient and integral part of the child's life, education on the principles of mainstreaming is needed for coaches, volunteers and educators.

Nonspecial Peers

A whole new type of educational program could be implemented to help the nonspecial peers and families understand the special child better. First, it needs to be understood that there is no law saying that the nonspecial family needs to be or is required to be involved in the mainstreaming process at all. The decision to mainstream is not theirs to make. They really have no say whatsoever about who is included in the mainstreaming activity and who is not. The federal government has mandated that the special individual has every right to participate in the activity of his or her choice and anyone or anything that acts to prevent that participation is discriminatory and in violation of the law. Including nonspecial families in the programming is strictly a volunteer effort to help them better understand the special child and his or her needs. In addition, the special family may feel more welcomed by nonspecial families when the fear of the unknown is eliminated.

It needs to be stressed to nonspecial families that special children are just like any of their own sons and daughters. They have feelings and emotions and can enjoy activities just like anyone else. They have friends and can participate together in the activity of their choice. The physically or mentally limiting condition they have is not "catching": It is not a disease; it is not a health hazard. It is just like one child's blue eyes or another child's black hair or another child's big stomach. The special child's place is in the community. Once the nonspecial family sees that these wonderful children are like any other child they meet on the street, the potential problem can be avoided. It's getting over that first hurdle that can be hard.

Individual Motivation

Another hurdle special children can encounter is their own emotional and spiritual conviction or lack of it.

There is no easy answer to the dilemma of what to tell a special child that will make him or her feel better. There must be something inside of each special child to want to do this. A child must be willing to face the big challenges involved and willing to work at resolving differences that may arise on the playing field — after all, they will come up, like it or not.

Certainly counselors and resource persons can help ease the transition for the child. They'll be there to answer questions and discuss fears that the special child may have. But there are some things that can be done to further help the special child feel more at ease.

The buddy system can be used, pairing individuals — one special and one nonspecial — to experience things together. Individuals with similar interests, hobbies or experiences might be paired together for better integration. One can lean on the other for support and strength, and the two together can ask and answer questions that will arise in the course of their time together.

Children can be grouped by interests. Instead of having just one support person in the form of a buddy, using a group for support may be useful. Group dynamics are much stronger than individual efforts and groups can better integrate the special child into the environment.

If the special child is still not at ease, and does not want to join a group or buddy system, there are still some things that can be done to ease the transition. The special child may just want to observe an activity a few times to be a part of it without being a total participant. The child might initially be assigned a special role to play on the team—such as scorekeeper, umpire or referee, or coach's "junior assistant"—until he or she feels comfortable enough to join the activity.

In any instance, it is initially important not to push children into something they may not really want to do, but at the same time, don't leave the special child out. It is important to encourage children to participate. Once they see that they *can do it*, they'll never want to stop.

Chapter Six

SPECIAL OLYMPICS

With most any living, breathing person, there is a thrill and enthusiasm for human competition. We can only practice for so long before we begin yearning to test our skills against others. It is a natural instinct to see how we "measure up" against our peers.

The child with mental retardation is no different in this respect. The companionship, the titillation, the thrill, the excitement of human competition is sought out by all challenged indivduals.

Therefore, this chapter provides information about Special Olympics International.

The following information is provided by SOI:

PHILOSOPHY

Mission
To provide year-round sports training and athletic competition in a variety of Olympic-type sports for children and adults with mental retardation, giving them continuing opportunities to develop physical fitness, demonstrate courage, experience joy and participate in the sharing of gifts, skills and friendship with their families, other Special Olympics athletes and the community.

Philosophy
Special Olympics is founded on the belief that people with mental retardation can, with proper instruction and encouragement, learn, enjoy and benefit from participation in individual and team sports, adapted as necessary to meet the needs of those with special mental and physical limitations.

Special Olympics believes that consistent training is essential to the development of sports skills, and that competition among those of equal abilities is the most appropriate means of testing these skills, measuring progress and providing incentives for personal growth.

Special Olympics believes that through sports training and competition, people with mental retardation benefit physically, mentally, socially and spiritually; families are strengthened; and the community at large, both through participation and observation, is united in understanding people with mental retardation in an environment of equality, respect and acceptance.

Principles

To provide the most enjoyable, beneficial and challenging activities for athletes with mental retardation, Special Olympics operates worldwide in accordance with the following principles and beliefs:

• That the spirit of Special Olympics — skill, courage, sharing and joy — incorporates universal values that transcend all boundaries of geography, nationality, political philosophy, gender, age, race or religion.

• That the goal of Special Olympics is to help bring all persons with mental retardation into the larger society under conditions whereby they are accepted, respected and given a chance to become productive citizens.

• That, as a means of achieving this goal, Special Olympics encourages its more capable athletes to move from Special Olympics training and competition into school and community programs where they can compete in regular sports activities. The decision to leave Special Olympics or continue is the athlete's choice.

• That all Special Olympics activities — at the local, state, national and international levels — reflect the values, standards, traditions, ceremonies and events embodied in the modern Olympic movement, broadened and enriched to celebrate the moral and spiritual qualities of persons with mental retardation so as to enhance their dignity and self-esteem.

• That participation in Special Olympics training programs and competitive events is open to all people with mental retardation who are at least eight years old, regardless of the degree of their disability.

• That comprehensive, year-round sports training is available to every Special Olympics athlete, conducted by well-qualified coaches in accordance with the standardized Sports Rules formulated and adopted by Special Olympics International; and that every athlete who participates in a Special Olympics sport will be trained in that sport.

• That every Special Olympics program includes sports events and activities that are appropriate to the age and ability of each athlete, from motor activities to the most advanced competition.

• That Special Olympics provides full participation for every athlete regardless of economic circumstance and conducts training and competition under the most favorable conditions possible, including facilities, administration, training, coaching, officiating and events.

• That Special Olympics gives each participant an equal chance to excel by basing competition in every event on accurate records of previous performance or trial heats and, when relevant, by grouping by age and gender.

• That, at every Awards Ceremony, in addition to the traditional medals for first, second and third places, athletes finishing from fourth to last place are presented a suitable place ribbon with appropriate ceremony.

• That, to the greatest extent possible, Special Olympics activities will be run by and involve local volunteers, from school and college age to senior citizens, in order to create greater opportunities for public understanding of and participation with people with mental retardation.

• That, although Special Olympics is primarily a program of sports training and competition, efforts are made to offer, as an integral part of Special Olympics Games, a full range of artistic, social and cultural experiences such as dances, art exhibits, concerts, visits to historic sites, clinics, theatrical performances and similar activities.

• That the goal of Special Olympics in every nation is to develop organizations and conduct events at the community level. Countries which, because of specific economic, social or cultural circumstances may find it difficult to achieve this goal rapidly, may hold National Games on a regular basis to enhance the development of popular understanding and provide increased visibility for their citizens with mental retardation. All participating countries are invited to send a delegation to the Special Olympics World Games held every two years, alternating between Summer and Winter, provided that, in all cases Special Olympics standards are adhered to in the preparation of athletes and coaches for the Games.

• That the families of Special Olympics athletes are encouraged to play an active role in their community Special Olympics program, to share in the training of their athletes and to assist in the public education effort needed to create greater understanding of the emotional, physical, social and spiritual needs of people with mental retardation and their families.

• That Special Olympics encourages community, state and national sports programs, both professional and amateur, to include demonstrations by Special Olympics athletes as part of their major events.

• That Special Olympics activities take place in public, with full coverage by the media, so that athletes with mental retardation may reveal to the world those special qualities of the human spirit in which they excel — skill, courage, sharing and joy.

THE SPORTS

Special Olympics offers year-round training and competition in twenty-two Olympic-type sports to children and adults with mental retardation. Participation is open to anyone ages eight and up, and programs are designed to serve all ability levels.

Official Summer Sports

- Aquatics
- Athletics
- Basketball

- Bowling
- Equestrian
- Football (Soccer)
- Gymnastics
- Roller Skating
- Softball
- Volleyball

Official Winter Sports

- Alpine Skiing
- Cross Country Skiing
- Figure Skating
- Speed Skating
- Floor Hockey
- Poly Hockey

Demonstration Sports

- Canoeing
- Cycling
- Table Tennis
- Team Handball
- Tennis
- Powerlifting

UNIFIED SPORTS®

Unified Sports® is a pioneer program that combines approximately equal numbers of athletes with and without mental retardation, of similar age and ability, on teams that compete against other Unified Sports® teams. Unified Sports® is an important program because it expands sports opportunities for athletes seeking new challenges and dramatically increases inclusion in the community.

After two years of field testing, the Unified Sports® program was launched throughout the United States in 1989. Current sports include Basketball, Bowling, Distance running and walking, Football

(Soccer), Softball, Volleyball and Cycling with several others under-going field testing.

Unified Sports® is a unique and influential program because it:

- Brings together athletes with and without mental retardation in a setting where everybody is challenged to improve.
- Provides a valuable sports opportunity to individuals with mental retardation who are not presently involved in Special Olympics, especially those with mild retardation, and those in communities where there are not enough Special Olympics athletes to conduct team sports.
- Allows athletes to develop specific sports skills and prepares them for participation in other community sports.
- Increases public awareness of the spirit and skills of individuals with mental retardation.
- Builds self-esteem and sports ability in all athletes by ensuring that each participant plays an important, meaningful and valued role on the team.
- Enables Special Olympics athletes' families to participate as team members or coaches on Unified Sports® teams.

How It Works

A Special Olympics Unified Sports® program can be conducted in a variety of settings, including:

- A program organized by a Special Olympics group.
- A community or church sports program, such as an adult softball league or YMCA volleyball league.
- An interscholastic or intramural after-school league at the junior high or high school level.
- As part of the league system at a local bowling center.
- An independent league sponsored by business or civic groups.
- A program in cooperation with a local recreation and park association.

Athletes with mental retardation who participate in Unified Sports® may or may not be involved in the local Special Olympics programs. Athletes without mental retardation can be recruited from schools, corporations, civic groups or other community organizations. These athletes must be similar in age and skill level to the athletes with mental retardation who participate in the program.

Unified Sports® teams are coached by volunteer coaches who may attend a Special Olympics Coaches Training School in the appropriate sport. Teams may participate in Unified Sports® divisions at Special Olympics Area, Chapter and International Games.

MOTOR ACTIVITIES TRAINING PROGRAM

The Motor Activities Training Program (MATP) provides comprehensive motor activity and recreation training for people with severe mental retardation or multiple disabilities, with emphasis on training and participation rather than competition. MATP is part of the commitment by Special Olympics to offer sports training opportunities to individuals with mental retardation of all ability levels.

After five years of consultation with educators, physical therapists and recreation specialists, and after field testing in the United States and several other countries, MATP was launched in 1989. A comprehensive Motor Activities Training Program Guide has been developed to assist trainers.

How It Works

MATP trains participants in motor-based recreation activities and enables them to take part in a program which is appropriate to the age and ability of each individual. After a training period of at least eight weeks, participants may take part in a Special Olympics Training Day, giving each participant a chance to demonstrate his or her "personal best" in an activity and to be recognized for this accomplishment. The skills learned through MATP also enable people with severe disabilities to participate in community recreational activities with their nondisabled peers.

While the goal of MATP is not necessarily to prepare persons with severe disabilities to participate in sports, many MATP participants will gain the skills required to compete in certain Special Olympics sports.

MATP trains participants in seven basic motor skills designed to relate to specific sports. The skills also complement training by educators and therapists in daily living skills. MATP trains participants in:

- Mobility: Gymnastics
- Dexterity: Athletics
- Striking: Softball
- Kicking: Football (Soccer)
- Manual Wheelchair: Athletics
- Electric Wheelchair: Athletics
- Aquatics

MATP can be implemented through schools, group homes, residential facilities and other community-based settings. Training for volunteers is available through Special Olympics Motor Activities Training Schools conducted by local Special Olympics programs.

The previous information on Special Olympics International was created by The Joseph P. Kennedy, Jr. Foundation for the Benefit of Citizens with Mental Retardation. Reprinted with permission.

Special Olympics is a truly unique, fantastic and incredibly amazing event to attend. You can see the struggle of the human spirit — competing without reservation, without regard and without animosity — to just have fun, and, if it happens, to win. Remember the Special Olympics oath, "Let me win. But if I cannot win, let me be brave in the attempt."

For information on volunteering, upcoming events or schedules, contact Special Olympics International at (202) 628-3630, or write:

Special Olympics International
International Headquarters
1350 New York Avenue N.W.
Suite 500
Washington, DC 20005

GLOSSARY OF TERMS

Adaptive behavior: Skills needed by a child to function effectively and appropriately for his or her age in the school, family and community settings.

American Sign Language (ASL): A signing system that conveys general ideas or thoughts, has its own grammatical rules, and is considered by many to be a true language.

Appropriate: As in "appropriate setting," an educational or social involvement program that can meet the requirements of a special needs child.

Apraxia: Inability to move the muscles involved in speech or other voluntary acts.

Articulation: Movement the vocal tract makes during production of speech sounds; enunciation of words and vocal sounds.

Ataxia: A condition characterized by awkwardness of fine and gross motor movements, especially those involved with balance, posture and orientation in space. It is a type of cerebral palsy.

Athetosis: A condition in which there are sudden, involuntary, jerky, writhing movements, especially of the fingers and wrists. It is a type of cerebral palsy.

Atrophy: Degeneration of tissue, such as muscles or nerves.

Autism: A childhood psychosis characterized by extreme withdrawal, self stimulation, and cognitive and perceptual deficits.

Cerebral palsy: A condition characterized by paralysis, weakness, incoordination, and/or other motor dysfunction due to brain damage.

Chronological age (CA): A child's actual age, usually stated in years and months (for example, 11-2 means 11 years, 2 months old).

Congenital: Existing at birth.

Cystic fibrosis: An inherited disease characterized by chronic respiratory and digestive problems.

Developmental delay: A temporary delay in a child's development of a skill or characteristic. Often referred to as a maturational lag.

Diabetes: A hereditary or developmental problem of sugar metabolism caused by a failure of the pancreas to produce enough insulin. Diabetes mellitus is the most common type.

Diplegia: A condition in which the legs are paralyzed to a greater extent than the arms.

Double hemiplegia: A condition in which both halves of the body are paralyzed but, unlike in quadriplegia, the two sides are affected differently.

Down syndrome: A condition resulting from a chromosomal abnormality characterized by mental retardation and such physical signs as slanted-appearing eyes, flattened features, shortness and a tendency toward obesity. The three major types of Down's syndrome are trisomy 21, mosaicism and translocation.

Dysarthria: A condition in which brain damage causes impaired control of the muscles used in articulation.

Early intervention: The provision of special services at an early age for special needs children to avoid more severe problems in the future.

Educational disability: A specific, cognitive, physical or emotional problem that impedes the learning process to the extent that specially designed instruction is necessary for a child to learn effectively.

Emotional lability: Frequent changes of mood.

Encephalitis: An inflammation of the brain that can adversely affect a child's mental development.

Endogenous: Mental retardation caused by social or genetic factors.

Epilepsy: A disorder characterized by recurring attacks of motory, sensory or psychic malfunction with or without unconsciousness or convulsive movements.

Exceptional child: A child whose educational and social needs differ so significantly from those of his or her peers that specially designed intervention is necessary. This term encompasses students who have special educational abilities (gifted) as well as disabilities.

Exogenous: Mental retardation caused by brain damage.

Expressive language disabilities: Problems associated with the inability to express oneself verbally.

Fine motor coordination: The ability to use small muscle movements to accomplish tasks requiring precision such as writing, cutting or sewing.

Finger spelling: The spelling out of the English sign language alphabet by various finger positions on one hand.

Focal seizure: A partial seizure involving a discharge in a fairly circumscribed part of the brain and so causing a limited motor or sensory effect.

Grade-level equivalent: A form of expressing a child's test performance. A child who performs on a test at the 4.3 grade level has achieved at a level typical of an "average" student in the third month (November) of the fourth grade.

Grand mal seizure: A major motor seizure in which the individual loses consciousness, falls and undergoes a short period of muscle rigidity followed by involuntary muscle contractions.

Gross motor coordination: The ability to use large muscle movements in a coordinated, purposeful manner to engage in such activities as running, throwing and kicking.

Handicapped child: The term used in federal and state laws to designate a child who has a specific cognitive, physical or emotional disability to the extent that specifically designed intervention is necessary for him or her to learn effectively.

Hemiplegia: A condition in which one half (right or left side) of the body is paralyzed.

Hydrocephalus: A condition characterized by enlargement of the head due to excessive pressure of the cerebrospinal fluid.

Hyperactivity: A higher degree of inappropriate motor activity than is considered typical for a particular age group.

Hyporesponsive: Slow to respond; opposite of hyperactive or distractible; characteristic of some learning-disabled children.

Hypoxia: Deficiency in the amount of oxygen reaching the tissues of the body.

Impulsivity: The tendency to respond quickly without carefully considering the alternatives; responding without adequate reflection.

Independent level: The highest level of a task that a child can perform independently and relatively free of tension.

Individualized Educational Program (IEP): A written plan that a team of school staff, parents and the child, if appropriate, develops for a special needs student. It must include, at a minimum, the child's current educational strengths and weaknesses, goals and objectives, educational services, start-up dates for those services, and procedures for program evaluation.

Informal test: A nonstandardized evaluative measure usually designed by an individual for a particular situation or purpose.

Instructional level: The level at which a child should be taught a task either academically or socially.

Intelligence quotient (IQ): Score on an intelligence test for which 100 is the mean. Indicates a child's test performance relative to other children of the same age; determined by dividing mental age by chronological age and multiplying by 100.

Kinesthesis: The sensation of bodily movements as perceived through the muscles, tendons and joints; the feeling of movement.

Language disorder: A lag in the ability to understand and express ideas; a lag that puts linguistic skill behind an individual's development in other areas, such as motor, cognitive or social development.

Least restrictive environment: A standard established by Public Law 94-142 for special educational placement. A child who has an educational disability must be allowed to participate in as much of a regular program as is appropriate in view of his or her special needs. The law holds that children with special needs must not be separated from others who do not have disabilities any more than is educationally necessary.

Mainstreaming: Placing a child who has special needs in an instructional or social setting in which most of his or her peers do not have disabilities, in a manner that is socially and educationally beneficial to the child.

Meningitis: A bacterial or viral infection of the linings of the brain or spinal cord.

Mental age (MA): A form of expressing a child's performance on an intelligence test. A child who receives an MA of 8-4 has achieved a score comparable to an "average" child of 8 years, 4 months old.

Mental retardation: A condition in which the individual has below average intellectual functioning; both IQ and adaptive skills are considered as levels of the retardation. The levels of retardation are mild, moderate, severe and profound judged according to IQ results.

Minimal brain dysfunction: A term used to describe a child who shows behavioral but not neurological signs of brain injury.

"Mixed" cerebral palsy: A type of cerebral palsy in which several types, such as athetosis and spasticity, occur together.

Modeling: Showing or demonstrating to others how to perform a particular behavior; among the most effective instructional methods an educator can use with a special needs child.

Monoplegia: A condition in which only one limb is paralyzed.

Multiple sclerosis: A chronic, slowly progressive disease of the central nervous system in which there is a hardening or scarring of the protective myelin sheath of certain nerves.

Muscular dystrophy: A hereditary disease characterized by progressive weakness caused by degeneration of muscle fibers.

Myopathy: A weakening and wasting away of the muscle tissue in which there is no evidence of neurological disease or impairment.

Neurosis: A condition marked by anxiety and an inability to cope with inner conflicts.

Norm: The average score on a test received by a group to which an individual's score can be compared.

Occupational therapy: Treatment by an occupational therapist to improve an individual's ability to integrate different mental and motor processes in a purposeful and efficient manner.

Organic: Inherent, inborn; involving known neurological or structural abnormality.

Orthotics: A professional specialty concerned with restoring of lost function of body parts using braces and adaptive devices.

Paraplegia: A condition in which both legs are paralyzed.

Perception: An individual's ability to process stimuli meaningfully; the ability to organize and interpret sensory information.

Perceptual-motor match: A theory that motor development precedes sensory (especially visual) development.

Petit mal seizure: A seizure characterized by brief lapses in or clouding of consciousness; these occur more often than grand mal seizures.

Phenylketonuria (PKU): A metabolic genetic disorder caused by the body's inability to convert phenylalanine to tyrosine; an accumulation of this phenylalanine results in brain dysfunction.

Phocomelia: A deformity in which the limbs of an infant are very short or missing completely, with the hands and feet attached directly to the torso; a syndrome commonly resulting from maternal use of the drug thalidomide during pregnancy.

Physical therapy: Treatment by physical and mechanical means to improve an individual's motor skills and increase the strength and endurance of body parts.

Placement: The setting in which a special needs child receives instruction.

Poliomyelitis: Also known as polio or infantile paralysis, an infectious disease that attacks the nerve tissue in the spinal cord and brain.

Prosthetics: A professional specialty concerned with replacing missing body parts with artificial substitutes (prostheses).

Psychosis: A major mental disorder, exhibited in seriously disturbed behavior and lack of contact with reality; childhood schizophrenia and autism are forms of psychosis.

Public Law 94-142 (P.L. 94-142): The Education for All Handicapped Children Act, which contains a mandatory provision stating that in order to receive funds under the act, every school system in the nation must make provision for a free appropriate public education for every child age three through twenty-one regardless of the type and severity of the handicap.

Quadriplegia: A condition in which all four limbs are paralyzed.

Receptive language disabilities: Difficulties that derive from the inability to understand spoken language.

Related services: Support services needed by a child to benefit from special placement (such as speech therapy, psychological counselling or special transportation).

Residential placement: A placement, usually arranged and paid for by a state agency or by the parents, where a child with special needs resides and typically receives academic and social instruction.

Resource teacher: Typically provides services for special needs children and their teacher within one setting, usually a school. The resource teacher assesses the particular needs of the children, sometimes teaches them individually or in small groups, and uses any special methods or materials that are necessary. The resource teacher consults with the regular educators and support staff, advising on instruction and management of special needs children in or out of the classroom and demonstrating instructional techniques.

Rheumatoid arthritis: A systematic disease with major symptoms involving the muscles and joints.

Rubella (German measles): A serious viral disease which is likely to cause a deformity in the fetus if it occurs during the first trimester of pregnancy.

Schizophrenia: Psychotic behavior manifested by loss of contact with reality, bizarre thought processes and inappropriate actions.

Scoliosis: Curvature of the spine; either congenital or acquired from poor posture, disease, or muscle weakness due to certain conditions such as cerebral palsy or muscular dystrophy.

Section 504: A federal civil rights law passed in 1973 to eliminate discrimination against people with disabilities in federally funded programs. Requires that special needs children receive educational services and opportunities equal to those provided to other children.

Seizure: A sudden alteration of consciousness, usually accompanied by motor activity and/or sensory phenomena; caused by an abnormal discharge of electrical energy in the brain.

Self-help skills: Skills related to the care of oneself such as eating, dressing and grooming.

Sign language: A manual system of "speaking" in which there is sometimes similarity between the hand configurations of each gesture and the meaning it represents.

Social-skills training: Instruction and activities designed to develop skills needed to interact appropriately with others.

Spasticity: A condition in which there are sudden involuntary contractions of the muscles, causing voluntary movements to be difficult and inaccurate; a type of cerebral palsy.

Special education: Specialized instruction for children who have educational disabilities based on a comprehensive evaluation. The instruction may occur in a variety of settings but must be precisely matched to their educational needs and adapted to their learning style.

Speech and language therapy: An individualized program of instruction and exercises provided by a speech therapist and designed to correct or improve speech disorders or problems of language usage.

Speech disorder: Indicated in oral communication that exhibits poor or abnormal use of the vocal apparatus; is unintelligible or so inferior that it draws attention to itself and causes anxiety, feelings of inadequacy or inappropriate behavior in the speaker.

Status epilepticus (status seizures): A condition in which an individual has continuous seizures.

Stuttering: Speech characterized by abnormal hesitations, prolongations and repetitions; may be accompanied by facial grimaces, gestures, or other bodily movements indicative of a struggle to speak, anxiety, blocking of speech, or avoidance of speech.

Tremor cerebral palsy: A type of cerebral palsy characterized by rhythmic, involuntary movement of certain muscles.

Tuberculosis: An infectious disease potentially causing tissue destruction in many organ systems, particularly the lungs.

Visual-motor integration: The ability to perceive visual images and reproduce them with a motor response (for example, swinging a bat at a ball and hitting it).

RESOURCES

A good general reference book for people with disabilities, or anyone working with children with disabilities, is *The Accessible Living Sourcebook*, Betterway Books.

The following organizations can provide a wide variety of information concerning many sports that they endorse or their members participate in.

American Athletic Association of the Deaf (AAAD)
1134 Davenport Dr.
Burton MI 48529
(313) 239-3962

National Handicapped Sports & Recreation Association
4405 East-West Highway
Bethesda MD 20814
(301) 652-7505

National Wheelchair Athletic Association (NWAA)
3617 Betty Dr.
Suite S
Colorado Springs CO 80907
(719) 597-8330

Special Olympics International (SOI)
1350 New York Ave. NW
Suite 500
Washington DC 20005
(202) 628-3630

United States Amputee Athletic Association (USAAA)
P.O. Box 210709
Nashville TN 37221
(615) 662-2323

United States Association for Blind Athletes (USABA)
33 N. Institute St.
Brown Hall, Suite 015
Colorado Springs CO 80903
(719) 630-0422

United States Cerebral Palsy Athletic Association (USCPAA)
34518 Warren Rd.
Suite 264
Westland MI 48185
(313) 425-8961

United States Les Autres Sports Association (USLASA)
1101 Post Oak Rd.
Suite 9-486
Houston TX 77056
(713) 521-3737

SPECIFIC SPORTS
Archery

National Archery Association of the United States
1750 E. Boulder St.
Colorado Springs CO 80909-5778
(719) 578-4576

NWAA NGB Chairperson
Sister Kenny Institute
800 E. Twenty-Eighth St. at Chicago Ave.
Minneapolis MN 55407
(617) 874-5712

Basketball

Amateur Basketball Association of the United States of America
(ABAUSA)
1750 E. Boulder St.
Colorado Springs CO 80909
(719) 632-7687

Federation Internationale de Basketball Amateur (FIBA)
19 Rugendastrasse
800 Munich 71, Germany

National Wheelchair Basketball Association (NWBA)
    % Dr. Stan Labanowich
    110 Seaton Building
    University of Kentucky
    Lexington KY 40506
    (606) 257-1623

Beep Baseball

Dr. Ed Bradley, President
    National Beep Baseball Association (NBBA)
    9623 Spencer Highway
    LaPorte TX 77571

Boating

American Canoe Association
    P.O. Box 1900
    Newington VA 22122
    (703) 550-7523
Adaptive Rowing Advisory Committee to the US Rowing Association
    % Richard Tobin
    St. Aubin Rowing Club
    11 Hall Place
    Exeter NH 03833
    (603) 778-0315
Philadelphia Rowing Program for the Disabled
    % Dolly Driscoll
    2601 Pennsylvania Ave. Apt. 146
    Philadelphia PA 19141
    (215) 765-2170
American Wheelchair Sailing Association (AWSA)
    Freedom Foundation
    512 Thirteenth St.
    Newport Beach CA 92663
    (714) 675-5427

Bowling

American Bowling Congress (ABC)
  5301 S. Seventy-Sixth St.
  Greendale WI 53129
  (414) 421-6400
American Wheelchair Bowling Association, Inc.
  Daryl L. Pfister, Executive Secretary
  N54 W15858 Larkspur Lane
  Menomonee Falls WI 53051
  (414) 781-6876
American Blind Bowling Association
  % Ron Beverly
  77 Bame Ave.
  Buffalo NY 14215
  (716) 836-1472

Cycling

United States Cycling Federation (USCF)
  1750 E. Boulder St.
  Colorado Springs CO 80909
  (719) 578-4581

Fencing

United States Fencing Association (USFA)
  1750 E. Boulder St.
  Colorado Springs, CO 80909
  (719) 578-4511
International Stoke Madeville Games Federation (ISMGF)
  Wheelchair Fencing Division
  Draadzegge 14
  2318 zm Leiden
  Netherlands

Field

The Athletic Congress of the USA (TAC)
P.O. Box 120
Indianapolis IN 46202
(317) 638-9155

International Amateur Athletic Federation (IAAF)
3 Hans Crescent, Knightsbridge
London SW1 0LN
U.K.

Fishing

Capable Partners
7320 Oxford St.
St. Louis Park MN 55426
(612) 938-5625

National Association of Handicapped Outdoor Sportsman, Inc.
(NAHOS)
R.R. 6, Box 25
Centralia IL 62801
(618) 985-3579

Physically Challenged Outdoorsman's Association
3006 Louisiana Ave.
Cleveland OH 44109

Floor Hockey

Walter Jackson, Director of Floor Hockey
San Diego Special Olympics
5384 Linda Vista Rd.
San Diego CA 92110
(619) 574-7589

Football

Santa Barbara Recreation Department
P.O. Box Drawer P-P
Santa Barbara CA 93102
(805) 962-1474

Goal Ball

USABA Sports Director for Goal Ball
　Stephen Kearney, Director of Athletics
　Oklahoma School for the Blind
　Box 309
　Muskogee OK 74401
　(918) 682-6641

Golf

National Amputee Golf Association (NAGA)
　Bob Wilson, Executive Director
　P.O. Box 1228
　Amherst NY 03031
　(603) 673-1135
Project FORE
　John Klein, PGA, Director of Golf
　5830 Wolff Court
　La Mesa CA 92042
　(619) 594-6699

Gymnastics

United States Gymnastics Federation (USGF)
　201 S. Capitol Ave.
　Indianapolis IN 46225
　(317) 237-5050
AIM (Adventures in Movement)
　945 Danbury Rd.
　Dayton OH 45420
　(513) 294-4611

Horseback Riding

American Horse Shows Association (AHSA)
　201 S. Capitol Ave.
　Suite 430
　Indianapolis IN 46225
　(317) 237-5252

North American Riding for the Handicapped Association (NARHA)
Bill Scebbi, Executive Director
Box 33150
Denver CO 80202
(303) 452-1212

Ice Skating

United States Figure Skating Association (USFSA)
20 First St.
Colorado Springs CO 80906
(719) 635-5200

United States International Speed Skating Association, Inc.
(USISSA)
17060 Patricia Lane
Brookfield WI 53005
(800) 334-7981

Skating Association for the Blind and Handicapped (SABAH)
% Sibley's Boulevard Mall Store
Niagara Falls Blvd.
Amherst NY 14226
(716) 833-2994

Lawn Bowling

ISMGF Chairman for Wheelchair Bowls
Mr. Roy Dunbar
17 Grenville Green
Aylesbury
Bucks HP21 8PP
U.K.

Quad Rugby

United States Quad Rugby Association
Brad Mickelson
2418 West Fallcreek Ct.
Grand Forks ND 58201
(701) 772-1961

Racquetball

American Amateur Racquetball Association (AARA) & National
Wheelchair Racquetball Association (NWRA)
815 N. Weber
Suite 203
Colorado Springs CO 80903
(719) 635-5396
United States Wheelchair Racquet Sports Association (USWRSA)
Chip Parmelly
1941 Viento Verano Dr.
Diamond Bar CA 91765
(714) 861-7312

Road Racing

The Athletic Congress of the USA (TAC)
P.O. Box 120
Indianapolis IN 46202
(317) 638-9155
The International Wheelchair Road Racers Club (IWRRC)
30 Myano Lane
Stamford CT 06902
(203) 967-2231
Achilles Track Club
9 E. Eighty-Ninth St.
New York NY 10128
(212) 967-9300

Roller Skating

U.S. Amateur Confederation of Roller Skating
1500 S. Seventieth St.
P.O. Box 6579
Lincoln NE 68506
(402) 483-7551

Federation Internationale de Roller Skating
   Gaylingstrasse 5
   7800 Zurich
   Switzerland

Rugball

Joe Millage, Program Coordinator
   Variety Village
   3701 Danforth Ave.
   Scarborough, Ontario M1N 2G2
   Canada

Showdown

Canadian Blind Sports Association
   333 River Rd.
   Ottawa, Ontario K1L 8H9
   Canada

Skiing

National Handicapped Sports & Recreation Association (NHSRA)
   4405 East-West Highway
   Bethesda MD 20814
   (301) 652-7505
United States Ski Association (USSA)
   1750 E. Boulder St.
   Colorado Springs CO 80909
   (719) 578-4600
American Blind Skiing Foundation
   610 S. William St.
   Mt. Prospect IL 60056
   (312) 353-4292

National Amputee Skiers Association (NASA)
3738 Walnut Ave.
Carmichael CA 95608

Three Track Ski
Box 1260, Station Q
Toronto, Ontario M4T 2P4
Canada

Sledge Hockey

Ottawa-Carleton Sledge Hockey & Ice Picking Association
46 Nestow Dr.
Nepean, Ontario K2G 3X8
Canada

Alberta Sledge Hockey & Ice Picking Association
20 Horner Ct., NE
Medicine Hat, Alberta T1C 1M1
Canada

Variety Village
3701 Danforth Ave.
Scarsborough, Ontario M1N 2G2
Canada

Soccer

United States Soccer Federation (USSF)
1750 E. Boulder St.
Colorado Springs CO 80909
(719) 578-6400

Soccer Association for Youth (SAY)
P.O. Box 921
Cincinnati OH 45201
(513) 351-SAY1

Amputee Soccer International
P.O. Box 7161
Seattle WA 98177
(206) 296-0348

Softball

Amateur Softball Association (ASA)
2801 NE Fiftieth St.
Oklahoma City OK 73111
(405) 424-5266

National Wheelchair Softball Association (NWSA)
Jon Speake, Commissioner
P.O. Box 22478
Minneapolis MN 55422
(612) 437-1792

Swimming

United States Swimming, Inc. (USS)
1750 E. Boulder St.
Colorado Springs CO 80909
(719) 578-4578

United States Swimming
Adapted Swimming Committee
Libby Anderson, Chairperson
4660 Natalie Dr.
San Diego CA 92115

Table Tennis

United States Table Tennis Association
1750 E. Boulder St.
Colorado Springs CO 80909
(719) 578-4583

American Wheelchair Table Tennis Association (AWTTA)
NWAA NGB Chairperson
166 Haase Ave.
Paramus NJ 07652

Team Handball

United States Team Handball Federation (USTHF)
1750 E. Boulder St.
Colorado Springs CO 80909
(719) 578-4582

Tennis

United States Tennis Association (USTA)
1212 Avenue of the Americas
New York NY 10036
(212) 302-3322

USTA Center for Educational & Recreational Tennis
729 Alexander Rd.
Princeton NJ 08540
(609) 452-2580

National Foundation of Wheelchair Tennis (NFWT)
Brad Parks, Executive Director
940 Calle Amancer, Suite B
San Clemente CA 92672
(714) 361-6811

Tennis Association for the Mentally Retarded (TAMR)
Kathy Wistert, President
2100 Wetstone Ct.
Thousand Oaks CA 91362
(805) 492-3753

United States Deaf Tennis Association (USDTA)
Gallaudet College
P.O. Box 1986
Washington DC 20002
(202) 651-5688

Track

The Athletic Congress of the USA (TAC)
P.O. Box 120
Indianapolis IN 46202
(317) 638-9155

International Amateur Athletic Federation (IAAF)
3 Hans Crescent, Knightsbridge
London SW1 0LN
U.K.

Volleyball

United States Volleyball Association (USVBA)
1750 E. Boulder St.
Colorado Springs CO 80909
(719) 632-5551
Ontario Wheelchair Sports Association
333 River Rd.
Ottawa, Ontario K1L 8H9
Canada
(613) 741-2463

Wrestling

U.S.A. Wrestling (USAW)
225 S. Academy
Colorado Springs CO 80910
(719) 597-8333

BIBLIOGRAPHY

Adams, R.C.; Daniel, A.N.; McCubbin, J.A; and Rullman, L. 1982. *Games, sports and exercises for the physically handicapped*. 3d ed. Philadelphia: Lea & Febiger.

American Amateur Racquetball Association. 1987. *Official Rule Book*. Colorado Springs: AARA.

Anderson, E.H., ed. 1986, Wheelchair team handball. *Team Handball USA*, May.

Anderson, L. 1988. Swimming to win. In *Training guide to cerebral palsy sports*, ed. J.A. Jones. Champaign, Ill.: Human Kinetics.

Andrews, M. 1981. Row cat mitts. *Sports 'N Spokes*. 7(1):6.

Axelson, P. 1986. Adaptive technology for skiing. *Palaestra*. 2(2):45-50.

Axelson, P. 1984. Sit skiing. *Sports 'N Spokes*. 9(5):28-31.

Bieber, N. 1988. Training riders for competition. In *Training Guide to Cerebral Palsy Sports*, ed. J.A. Jones 137-143. Champaign, Ill.: Human Kinetics.

Brenner, R. 1980. Rabcan bankshot basketball gives basketball a whole new challenge. *Sports 'N Spokes*. 6(1):8-9.

Cecotti, F. 1982. Electronic fishing reels: A fishing reel for the severely disabled. *Sports 'N Spokes*. 8(2):18-19.

Cowart, J. 1985. An adapted bowling device for severely disabled individuals. *Palaestra*. 2(1):38-39.

Cowart, J. 1978. Teacher-made adapted devices for archery, badminton, and table tennis. *Practical Pointers*. 1(13).

Cowen, L.; Sibille, J.; and O'Riain, M.D. 1984. Motor soccer: The electric connection. *Sports 'N Spokes*. 10(4):43-44.

Crase, N.; Schmid, R.; and Robbins, S. 1987. Pedal power. *Sports 'N Spokes*. 12(5):27-30.

Dimsdale, A. 1988. Quad rugby competition. *Sports 'N Spokes*. 14(1):18-19.

Dimsdale, A., and Beck, A. 1988. The first US quad rugby championships. *Sports 'N Spokes*. 14(2):28-30.

Dwight, M.P. 1988. *What is team handball?* Mt. Pleasant, Mich.: Michigan Special Olympics.

Eagleson, J. 1988. Growing programs help disabled enjoy freedom on the water. *Soundings*, Jan. 15-19.

Goodin, G. 1983. Quad rugby: Sometimes known as murder ball. *Sports 'N Spokes.* 9(4):26-27.

Grosse, S. 1985. It's a wet and wonderful world! *Palaestra.* 2(1):14-17.

Hamilton, B. 1988. Playoff determines blister bowl champ. *Sports 'N Spokes.* 13(5):29-30.

Hood, C.; Ryan, S.; Kelly, M.; and Bialowas, S. 1988. Improved picks help performance. *Sports 'N Spokes.* 14(4):50.

Jones, J.; Todd, T.; and Tetreault, P. 1987. U.S. Olympic festival: Disabled athlete participation. *Palaestra.* 4(1):48-53,64.

Jones, J.A. 1988. General considerations for field events. In *Training guide to cerebral palsy sports*, ed. J.A. Jones, 97-106. Champaign, Ill.; Human Kinetics.

Jones, J.A. 1988. To float or not to float. In *Training guide to cerebral palsy sports*. ed. J.A. Jones. Champaign, Ill.: Human Kinetics.

Jones, J.A. 1988. Wheelchair boccia. In *Training guide to cerebral palsy sports*. ed. J.A. Jones, 173-181. Champaign, Ill.: Human Kinetics.

Jones, J.A., and Mushett, M. 1984. Wheelchair soccer. In *Training guide to cerebral palsy sports*. ed. J.A. Jones. Champaign, Ill.: Human Kinetics.

Jones, M.B. 1988. Archery. In *Training guide to cerebral palsy sports* ed. J.A. Jones, 145-151 Champaign, Ill.: Human Kinetics.

Joswick, R.; Kittredge, M.; McCowan, L.; McParland, J.; and Woods, G. 1986. *Aspects and answers: A manual for therapeutic horseback riding programs.* Battle Creek, Mich.: Cheff Center.

Kearney, S., and Copeland, R. 1979. Goal ball. *Journal of Health, Physical Education, Recreation and Dance.* 50(7):24-26.

Kegel, B. 1985. Sport and recreation for those with lower limb amputations or impairments. *Journal of Rehabilitation Research and Development*, Clinical Supplement No. 1. Washington, D.C.: Veterans Administration.

Klein, J. 1979. "Handicapped" is a state of mind. *PGA Magazine*. 13(1):24-25.

LaMere, T., and Labanowich, S. 1984. The history of sport wheelchairs — Part 1: The development of the basketball wheelchair. *Sports 'N Spokes*. 9(6):6-8, 10, 11.

Lewis, J. 1988. Coaching slalom. In *Training guide to cerebral palsy sports*, ed. J.A. Jones. Champaign, Ill.: Human Kinetics.

Lippert, L. 1982. The quad slalom: Why not obstacles? *Sports 'N Spokes*. 8(3):19.

Longo, P. 1980. Golf. *Sports 'N Spokes*. 6(4):15-17.

Mastro, J.V. 1986. Wrestling: A viable sport for the visually impaired. *Journal of Health, Physical Education, Recreation and Dance*. 57(9):61-64.

McBee, F. 1981. The 1st world wheelchair marathon championship. *Sports 'N Spokes*. 6(6):21-23.

Millage, J.G., and Longmuir, P.E. 1987. Rugball — A sport for everyone. *Sports 'N Spokes*. 13(2):63-64.

Montelione, T., and Mastro, J.V. 1985. Beep baseball. *Journal of Health, Physical Education, Recreation and Dance*. 56(6):60-61, 65.

National Beep Baseball Association. 1987. *NBBA guide*. La Porte, Tex.: NBBA.

National Wheelchair Athletic Association. 1988. *Official NWAA rules*. Colorado Springs: NWAA.

National Wheelchair Basketball Association. 1986. *National wheelchair basketball tournament program*. Chicago, Ill.: National Wheelchair Basketball Association.

Nesbit, J. 1986. *The international directory of recreation-oriented assistive device sources*. Marina del Rey, Calif.: Lifeboat Press.

Nobels, B. 1981. Rhythmic Gymnastics. *Sports 'N Spokes*. 7(2):15-16.

Nordhaus, R.S.; Kantrowitz, M.; and Siembieda, W.J. 1984. *Acces-*

sible fishing: A planning handbook. Santa Fe, N. Mex.: New Mexico Natural Resources Department.

Nunnenkamp, B. 1976. Bowling from a wheelchair. *Sports 'N Spokes.* 2(2):17-19.

Special Olympics. 1988. *Official Special Olympics rules.* Washington, D.C.: Special Olympics.

Special Olympics. 1988. *Official Special Olympics winter sports rules.*Washington D.C.: Special Olympics.

Ontario Wheelchair Sports Association. 1982. *Introduction to table tennis.* Toronto: Ontario Wheelchair Sports Association.

Ontario Wheelchair Sports Association. 1982. *Introduction to track and field.* Toronto: Ontario Wheelchair Sports Association.

Ontario Wheelchair Sports Association. 1981. *Introduction to volleyball.* Toronto: Ontario Wheelchair Sports Association.

Orr, R.E., and Sheffield, J. 1979. Racquetball. *Sports 'N Spokes.* 5(2):6-7.

Owens, D. 1984. *Teaching golf to special populations.* Champaign, Ill.: Human Kinetics.

Radocy, B. 1987. Upper extremity prosthetics: Consideration and designs for sports and recreation. *Clinical Prosthetics and Orthotics.* 11(3): 131-153.

Rapport, A. 1982. Sledge hockey: The alternative to ice hockey for the disabled. *Sports 'N Spokes.* 8(4):24-25.

Rich, S.M. 1987. Beep baseball: A game of challenge. *Palaestra.* 4(1):40-43.

Roper, P., and Roberts, P. 1988. Soccer strategies for the beginning coach and team. In *Training guide to cerebral palsy sports,* ed. J.A. Jones. Champaign, Ill.: Human Kinetics.

Schwandt, D. 1980. Para-bike. *Sports 'N Spokes.* 6(4):18-19, 21.

Shasby, G., and Lyttle, J. 1981. Row, row, row your boat. *Sports 'N Spokes.* 7(1):5,7.

Stephenson, D., and Mushett, M. 1988. Wheelchair team handball. In *Training guide to cerebral palsy sports.* ed. J.A. Jones. Champaign, Ill.: Human Kinetics.

Tetreault, J., and Tetreault, P. 1988. Training techniques for track events. In *Training guide to cerebral palsy sports*. ed. J.A. Jones. Champaign, Ill.: Human Kinetics.

Thompson, G. 1984. Quadriplegic tennis? You bet!!! *Sports 'N Spokes*. 10(2):8.

United States Association for Blind Athletes. 1986. *USABA Official Sports Rules*. Beach Haven Park, N.J.: USABA.

United States Cerebal Palsy Athletic Association. 1988. *Classification and Sports Rules Manual*. Westland, Mich.: USCPAA.

United States Tennis Association. 1986. *Directory of tennis programs for the disabled*. Princeton, N.J.: USTA.

Webel, G., and Balicki, J. 1985. Adaptive boating for people with disabilities. *Trends*. 22(2):41-45.

Wilson, B. 1988. Amputee golf . . . We play with what we have left! *Palaestra*. 4(2):33-34.

Windover, R. 1988. Sledge hockey tournament. *Sports 'N Spokes*. 14(1):17-18.

Yarusso, G. 1982. Ridin' in the Ring: A look at disabled equestrians. *Paraplegia News*, Nov. 32-35.

INDEX

S

Schizophrenia; defined, 109
Scissor kicks, 41
Scoliosis; defined, 109
Section 504; defined, 109
Seizure; defined, 109
Self-help skills; defined, 110
Sensory impairments, 6-8; endogenous causes, 6; exogenous causes, 6; hearing loss, 6-7; vision loss, 7-8
Shoulder presses, 42, 47
Shoulder shrugs, 39
Shoulder stretches, 39
Shoulder touches, 39
Showdown, 70
Sickle cell anemia; defined, 15
Side arm presses, 45
Side dives, 47
Sign language, 28-32; defined, 110; encouragement, 32; finger language, 29-30; guidelines, 31-32; history, 28; types, 29-30; universality, 29
Simplified language structure, 19-22
Sitting leg pulls, 46
Sit-ups, modified, 41
Skating, ice, 64-65
Skating, roller, 68
Skiing, 70-72
Slalom, 72
Sledge hockey, 73
Soccer, 73-75
Soccer, motor, 66
Social-skills training; defined, 110
Softball, 75-76
Spasticity; defined, 110
Special education; defined, 110
Special Olympics, 95-102; mission, 95; Motor Activities Training Program (MATP), 101-102; philosophy, 95-96; principles, 96-98; sports, 98-99; Unified Sports, 99-101

Speech and language therapy; defined, 110
Speech disorders, 9-10; defined, 110
Spina bifida; defined, 13
Spinal cord injuries; defined, 13
Sports, 49-83
Status epilepticus (status seizures); defined, 110
Stuttering; defined, 110
Swan dives, 47
Swimming, 76-78

T

Table tennis, 78
Team handball, 78-80
Tennis, 80
Tennis, table, 78
Tippy-toes, 44
Toe paddles, 42
Toe touches, 40
Toss darts, 80-81
Track, 81-82
Tremor cerebral palsy; defined, 110
Tuberculosis; defined, 110
Twisters, 40-41

U

Unified Sports, 99-101

V

Vision loss, 7-8
Visual-motor integration; defined, 110
Volleyball, 82-83

W

Wall pushes, 47
Warm-up exercises, 39-42
Wrestling, 83
Wrist fan curls, 40
Wrist twists, 40

Z

Zero reject model, 86-87

More Books in The Parent's Guide *Series*

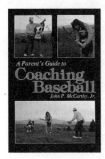 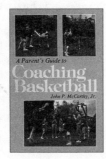 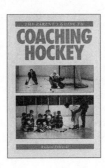 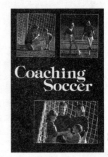

Your influence as a coach or teacher can give children (both yours and others) the greatest gifts of all: strong self-confidence and high self-esteem. *The Parent's Guide* series has nearly a dozen books full of helpful illustrations and step-by-step instructions on how to nurture and encourage children as they strive for success in sports and the arts. Plus, the friendly, familiar tone of each book will help both you and the child have fun as you learn.

The Parent's Guide to Coaching Baseball *#70076/128 pages/$7.95, paperback*

The Parent's Guide to Coaching Basketball *#70077/136 pages/$7.95, paperback*

The Parent's Guide to Coaching Football *#70078/144 pages/$7.95, paperback*

The Parent's Guide to Coaching Hockey *#70216/176 pages/$8.95, paperback*

The Parent's Guide to Coaching Soccer *#70079/136 pages/$8.95, paperback*

The Parent's Guide to Coaching Tennis *#70080/144 pages/$7.95, paperback*

The Parent's Guide to Coaching Skiing *#70217/144 pages/$8.95, paperback*

The Parent's Guide to Teaching Music *#70082/136 pages/$7.95, paperback*

The Parent's Guide to Band and Orchestra *#70075/136 pages/$7.95, paperback*

The Parent's Guide to Teaching Art: How to Encourage Your Child's Artistic Talent and Ability *#70081/184 pages/$11.95, paperback*

Use the order form below (photocopy acceptable) and save when you order two or more books!

- -

☐ **Yes!** I want the following books to help my child grow:

Book #	Brief title	Price
_____	_____	_____
_____	_____	_____
_____	_____	_____

Visa/MasterCard Orders Call TOLL-FREE
1-800-289-0963

*Add $3 postage and handling for one book; postage is FREE when you order 2 or more books.

Subtotal _____
Tax (Ohio residents only, 5.5%) _____
Postage & handling* _____
Total _____

Check enclosed $ _____ ☐ Visa ☐ MasterCard

Acct # _____ Exp. _____

Name _____ Signature _____

Address _____

City _____ State _____ Zip _____

Stock may be limited on some titles; prices subject to change without notice.
Mail to: Betterway Books, 1507 Dana Ave., Cincinnati, OH 45207

3131